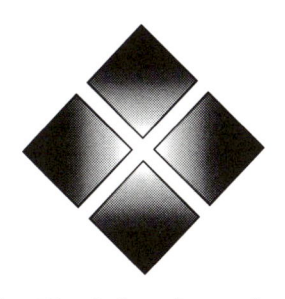

A Guide for the
Healthcare Professional

Informed Consent

Other Books in the Guide for the Healthcare Professional Series

Antitrust Law, by Jonathan P. Tomes, 1993

Environmental Law, by Jonathan P. Tomes, 1993

Fraud, Waste, Abuse and Safe Harbors, by Jonathan P. Tomes, 1993

EDI, by James J. Moynihan, 1993

Industry Regulation, by Jonathan P. Tomes, 1993

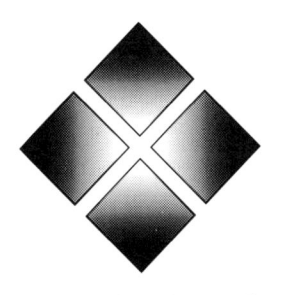

A Guide for the
Healthcare Professional

Informed Consent

Jonathan P. Tomes, J.D.

PROBUS PUBLISHING COMPANY
Chicago, Illinois
Cambridge, England

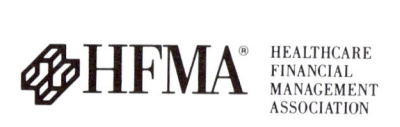

HFMA® HEALTHCARE FINANCIAL MANAGEMENT ASSOCIATION

KF
3827
.I5
T65
1993

© 1993, Probus Publishing Company

ALL RIGHTS RESERVED. No part of this publication may be reproduced, stored in a retrieval system, or transmitted by any means, electronic, mechanical, photocopying, recording, or otherwise, without the prior written permission of the publisher and the copyright holder.

This publication is designed to provide accurate and authoritative information in regard to the subject matter covered. It is sold with the understanding that the publisher is not engaged in rendering legal, accounting or other professional service.

Authorization to photocopy items for internal or personal use, or the internal or personal use of specific clients, is granted by PROBUS PUBLISHING COMPANY, provided that the US$7.00 per page fee is paid directly to Copyright Clearance Center, 27 Congress Street, Salem MA 01970, USA; Phone: 1-508-744-3350. For those organizations that have been granted a photocopy license by CCC, a separate system of payment has been arranged. The fee code for users of the Transactional Reporting Service is: 1-882198-08-5/93/$0.00 + $7.00.

ISBN 1-882198-08-5

Printed in the United States of America

BB

1 2 3 4 5 6 7 8 9 0

Table of Contents

Chapter 1	**What Is Informed Consent and Why Is It Important?**	1
	Introduction	1
	Battery—A Failure to Obtain Any Consent	2
	Failure to Obtain Informed Consent	3
	Conclusion	4
	Notes	5
Chapter 2	**Who May Consent?**	7
	Introduction	7
	Substituted Consent	8
	Emergency Exceptions	19
	Conclusion	22
	Notes	22
Chapter 3	**When Do You Need Informed Consent?**	27
	Introduction	27
	Treatment Requiring Consent	27
	Treatment Requiring Informed Consent	28
	Special Situations Requiring Informed Consent	32
	Conclusion	40
	Notes	40

Chapter 4	**How Do You Get Informed Consent?**	43
	Introduction	43
	How Much Information Must the Physician Disclose?	43
	What Is the Standard for Disclosure?	45
	Information to Be Disclosed	46
	What Need Not Be Disclosed	47
	The Therapeutic Privilege	48
	Emergency	49
	Conclusion	50
	Notes	50
Chapter 5	**Liability for Failure to Obtain Consent**	53
	Introduction	53
	Liability for Battery	53
	Liabilty for Failure to Obtain Informed Consent	54
	Facility Liability for a Practitioner's Failure to Obtain Consent	57
	Conclusion	59
	Notes	60
Chapter 6	**Federal Informed Consent Laws**	61
	Introduction	61
	Informed Consent for Research	61
	Other Federal Guidance	65
	Conclusion	66
	Notes	66
Chapter 7	**State Informed Consent Laws**	69
	Introduction	69
	Alabama	69
	Alaska	70
	Arizona	71

Contents

Arkansas	71
California	72
Colorado	72
Connecticut	73
Delaware	73
Florida	74
Georgia	75
Hawaii	76
Idaho	76
Illinois	77
Indiana	77
Iowa	78
Kansas	78
Kentucky	78
Louisiana	79
Maine	80
Maryland	81
Massachusetts	81
Michigan	82
Minnesota	82
Mississippi	83
Missouri	84
Montana	84
Nebraska	84
Nevada	85
New Hampshire	85
New Jersey	86
New Mexico	86
New York	87
North Carolina	87
North Dakota	88
Ohio	89
Oklahoma	89

	Oregon	90
	Pennsylvania	90
	Rhode Island	91
	South Carolina	91
	South Dakota	92
	Tennessee	92
	Texas	93
	Utah	93
	Vermont	94
	Virginia	95
	Washington	95
	West Virginia	96
	Wisconsin	96
	Wyoming	97
	Conclusion	97
	Notes	97
Chapter 8	**Facility Consent Policy**	103
	Introduction	103
	Legally Sufficient Consent Policy	103
	Consent Forms	105
	Conclusion	109
	Notes	110
Appendix I	**Sample Consent Policy**	111
	Introduction	111
	Forms	111
	Procedure	113
Appendix II	**Sample Consent Forms**	121
Glossary		145
Bibliography		149
Index		151
About the Author		163

Chapter 1

What Is Informed Consent and Why Is It Important?

Introduction

Informed consent is a comparatively recent legal doctrine. It requires a physician to inform a patient of medical procedures and their consequences so the patient can make an informed decision whether to submit to the treatment or not. As recently as 1972, one court defined informed consent as "a negligence concept predicated on the duty of a physician to disclose to a patient information that will enable him to 'evaluate knowledgeably the options available and the risks attendant upon each' before subjecting that patient to a course of treatment."[1]

Although the concept of patient participation in medical decision making did not exist until the mid-twentieth century, at that time, the law began to recognize the right of patients to consent to medical procedures.[2] Judicial decisions establishing this doctrine early in this century arose from physicians' failure to get permission from their patients to perform surgery. The courts recognized the patients' right to be free from an unauthorized touching and allowed them to recover as if they had been the victim of a battery—an unconsented harmful or offensive touching.[3]

By the 1950s, the courts realized that actions alleging a lack of *informed* consent differed from those arising from a total lack of consent. A lack of informed consent is based on negligence—a failure to use due care—as opposed to a battery, which is an intentional act. Thus, courts separated cases involving failure to give patients adequate information upon which to make an informed decision regarding treatment alternatives from those in which no consent had been obtained at all.[4] The modern doctrine of informed consent rests on a negligence theory, i.e., a physician violates his duty to his patient if he withholds any facts that are necessary to form the basis of an intelligent consent by the patient to the proposed treatment.[5] Of course, even with informed consent, a physician may still be liable for medical malpractice—a failure to provide the quality of care required by law—if he or she performs the authorized treatment improperly.

Thus, consent cases can arise in one of two ways: in the original way, as a battery, for the performance of procedures different from or in excess of those to which the patient consented, or under the more recent negligence theory, where the physician performs the procedure to which his patient consented, but fails to disclose certain risks and results involved in the procedure and thereby fails to obtain informed consent.

Battery—A failure to obtain any consent

Because battery is an intentional tort—a civil wrong, entitling the victim to damages—the plaintiff need not prove that the physician was negligent in any manner. All the plaintiff must prove is that the physician touched the plaintiff without the patient's consent, as by performing an unauthorized operation. Even if the surgery proves to be 100 percent successful and the patient is better off from the procedure, the physician is liable for battery, because the patient need only prove an unauthorized touching.

From a plaintiff's perspective, bringing a battery case against a practitioner is preferable to bringing a negligence action. The physician has few defenses to a battery, and the plaintiff need not prove through expert testimony what the standard of care was and that the defendant's conduct fell below that standard. All the plaintiff must do is demonstrate that an unconsented touching occurred. Further, courts are more willing to award punitive damages in battery-based lawsuits than in ones predicated upon negligence.[6]

Failure to obtain informed consent

The doctrine of informed consent, however, is more than an unauthorized touching. It goes to the heart of the doctor-patient relationship, and its evolution reflects changes that have taken place in that relationship. The traditional elements of that relationship are:

1. The doctor has a special knowledge that affects the welfare of the patient

2. The patient relies on the doctor's skill for his or her welfare

3. The doctor has a special obligation and responsibility to use his skill to provide the most beneficial treatment possible to the patient

As stated above, more recent court decisions and statutes have recognized the patient's right to make the final determination as to the kind of treatment that is most beneficial and in his or her best interests. Thus, these laws add the following elements to the doctor-patient relationship:

1. The patient has the right to be the final arbiter of which healthcare treatment (including no treatment) is in his or her best interests
2. The patient relies upon the doctor's special knowledge and skill to determine the treatment that is in his or her best interests

This change or addition to patients' rights has expanded the doctor's responsibilities. The doctor not only has the responsibility to provide the proper care, he or she now also must provide the proper information to enable the patient to make the proper healthcare decision regarding alternate procedures and their attendant risks.

Thus, in informed consent cases based on negligence, the plaintiff must prove that the defendant breached a duty to disclose information and prove that the failure to adequately disclose that information harmed the patient. Such harm exists when disclosure of significant risks incidental to the treatment would have resulted in the patient deciding against undergoing the treatment.[7]

Conclusion

A knowledge of informed consent is becoming increasing important to healthcare providers. Practitioners are generally aware of the stringent standards of care they must follow in order to avoid liability for malpractice actions once treatment has begun. However, the informed consent doctrine confronts practitioners even before they begin treatment and may result in a lawsuit notwithstanding otherwise excellent medical care.[8] In addition, the American Hospital Association recently noted that informed consent problems have become more complicated.

> Advances in medical technology and heightened consumer awareness among patients are fueling a rise in some kinds of informed consent claims. And although such claims still make up a small percentage of total claims against most hospitals, experts say that attention to this area is warranted now more than ever.
>
> Further, plaintiff's attorneys are finding judges and juries more sympathetic to informed consent claims. This change in attitude should encourage hospitals to carefully scrutinize their informed consent processes, risk-management experts say.[9]

This book will help you ensure that your facility has a good informed consent policy to minimize liability for failure to obtain informed consent. In order to do so, the remainder of this book discusses who may consent, including substituted consent from parents or legal guardians when the patient cannot consent and the emergency exception when the delay in obtaining consent would harm the patient, when informed consent is necessary, how to obtain informed consent, and how to develop an informed consent policy.

Notes

1. Perna v. Pirozzi, 457 A.2d 431, 438 (N.J. 1983) (quoting Canterbury v. Spence, 464 F.2d 772, 780 (D.C. Cir. 1972), cert. denied, 409 U.S. 1064 (1972).

2. See Richard E. Shugrue & Kathyrn Linstromberg, "Practitioner's Guide to Informed Consent," *Creighton Law Review 24*, 880–82 (1990–91).
3. See e.g. Schloendorff v. Society of New York Hospital, 105 N.E. 92 (N.Y. 1914); Mohr v. Williams, 104 N.W. 12 (Minn. 1905).
4. Shugrue & Lindstromberg, "Practitioner's Guide," 882–83.
5. Salgo v. Leland Stanford Jr. Univ. Bd. of Trustees, 317 P.2d 170, 181 (Cal. Ct. App. 1957).
6. Barry R. Furrow, Sandra H. Johnson, Timothy S. Jost, & Robert L. Schwartz, *Health Law, Cases, Materials and Problems*, 2d ed. St. Paul, Minn.: West Publishing Co., 1991 (hereafter Health Law), 327.
7. Id., 345–46.
8. Practitioner's Guide, 881–2.
9. Terese Hudson, "Informed Consent Problems Become More Complicated," *Hospitals* 1991, 65: 6 (March 20, 1991), 38–40.

Chapter 2

Who May Consent?

Introduction

Healthcare providers often face the situation where the patient cannot consent because he or she is a minor, is incompetent, or is unconscious. In such situations, the facility must have a policy for substituted consent—obtaining consent from another person authorized to give consent—and for when the practitioner may proceed without consent in emergency situations.

Obviously, a competent adult patient may consent for him- or herself. In some cases, however, a physician or facility will find it difficult or impossible to obtain informed consent from the person in need of medical treatment. The person may be unconscious, may be an infant or young child, or may be conscious but incapable of understanding and evaluating the information about her medical treatment options for any number of reasons, such as severe pain, intoxication, or mental impairment. Also, time may not permit the attending physician to obtain informed consent if the need for medical treatment is urgent and any delay would endanger the patient.

Substituted consent

When the patient cannot give consent on his or her own behalf, healthcare providers must still obtain informed consent in the form of substituted consent or fall within an exception to the informed consent doctrine before providing medical treatment. Otherwise, they risk liability for battery or medical malpractice for failure to obtain informed consent. *Substituted consent* is consent or authorization from a person who the law recognizes as having the authority to give consent on behalf of the person receiving treatment. It is required for minors and for incompetent patients. In addition, the law implies consent in the case of emergencies, providing an exception to the informed consent doctrine.

Authorized persons

Whenever a healthcare provider cannot obtain informed consent from the person in need of medical treatment and an emergency does not justify the emergency exception discussed below, the provider must obtain informed consent from an *authorized person*—another person who the law authorizes to give consent on behalf of the person in need of medical treatment. When obtaining this substituted consent, the healthcare provider must disclose all information to the authorized person regarding the proposed medical treatment that would have been disclosed to the person in need of the treatment if that person had been able to give consent for him- or herself.

State statutes generally provide that substituted consent may be given by the following persons:

- A parent for a minor child or an adult child of unsound mind (defined as an inability, for whatever reason, to perceive all relevant facts related to one's condition and proposed treatment so as to make an intelligent decision)

- A married person for his or her spouse
- Any person temporarily standing *in loco parentis* (in place of the parent), whether formally serving as such or not, for any minor in his or her care; and any guardian for his or her ward
- In the absence of a parent, any adult, for his or her sibling
- In the absence of a parent, any grandparent, for his or her minor grandchild[1]

If no family member or guardian is willing or able to give substituted consent or if more than one person is authorized to give such consent and they disagree as to what, if any, medical treatment the practitioner may provide, the healthcare practitioner should seek a court order either authorizing treatment or appointing a guardian to do so.[2] A court order may also be necessary if the person authorized to give substituted consent refuses consent for medical or surgical treatment that the healthcare provider, in the exercise of professional medical judgment, believes is necessary.

Legal issues to consider regarding medical decision making for those unable to make their own decisions vary, depending on whether the person in need of medical treatment is a minor, is incompetent, or is incapacitated due to a condition requiring emergency or urgent care.

Minor patients

The United States Supreme Court has recognized that parents have a fundamental liberty interest in matters of family life, including how they raise and care for their children.[3] Accordingly, a healthcare provider must obtain consent from a parent of a minor before providing the child with any medical or surgical treatment, unless one of several exceptions applies.

In cases of medical emergency, when little or no time exists to discuss the risks of and alternatives to the proposed treatment and to obtain parental consent, consent is not necessary. See the discussion below as to what constitutes a medical emergency.

Rule of Sevens. Parental consent is also unnecessary when the law deems the minor in need of medical treatment to be competent to give informed consent on his or her own behalf. Under the so-called Rule of Sevens, minors under the age of seven years cannot give valid consent for medical treatment.[4] In the absence of a statute providing a different rule, the courts presume that children of that age or younger are incapable of understanding and appreciating the consequences of the proposed medical treatment and, therefore, could not give effective consent. The same presumption applies to minors between the ages of 7 and 14, except that minors in this category may rebut this presumption by showing that they are of sufficient intelligence and maturity to make their own medical treatment decisions and give informed consent on their own behalf. Once a minor reaches the age of 14 years, the law presumes that he or she is capable of giving informed consent unless someone shows that the minor lacks the requisite intelligence or maturity to do so.

Consent by minor. The influence of the Rule of Sevens has led to the enactment of consent laws in many states that specifically address a minor's capacity to consent. In these states, minors may give consent for their own medical treatment once they marry.[5] Once the minor has obtained this capacity to consent by marriage, divorce or annulment do not nullify it. Other events that may trigger a minor's capacity to consent are:

- Giving birth to a child[6]

- Graduating from high school[7]

- Becoming emancipated (the freeing of a minor from parental control)[8]

- Being on active duty with any branch of the United States armed forces[9]

A few states allow a minor to make his or her own medical decisions once the minor can show sufficient intelligence to "understand and appreciate the consequences of the proposed surgical or medical treatment or procedures."[10] In addition, many states allow minors to consent to treatment for specific medical conditions, such as pregnancy, sexually transmitted diseases and substance or alcohol abuse, regardless of age.[11]

Authorization by the state. Last, a healthcare provider may treat a child without parental consent when (1) the parents refuse to consent to medical treatment the healthcare provider, in the exercise of medical judgment, believes is necessary, and (2) the treatment is authorized by a court order or by a court-appointed guardian for the child. As a general proposition, parents are free to raise their children according to the dictates of their own consciences. However, parents are required by law to provide adequate food, clothing, shelter, education, and medical care for their children. If a child's parents fail to provide the child with these necessities, the state, through its *parens patriae* power (the role of the state as the guardian of persons under legal disability), may declare the child dependent or neglected and take custody of the child to ensure his or her needs are met.

Often parents refuse to consent to medical treatment for their child on the basis of religious beliefs. In several cases, parents have refused to allow a blood transfusion for their child because they believed infusion of blood or blood products would lead to their child's damnation.[12] In other cases, the parents' refusals were based on their belief that prayer was sufficient to treat their child's condition or that the use of medicine of any kind was forbidden by their faith.[13] Under most circumstances, the court will find that the state's interest in preserving the child's life outweighs the parents' rights to privacy and to the free exercise of their religion.

Whether a court will assert the state's *parens patriae* power to authorize treatment of a child over parental objection depends, in part, on its determination of the best interests of the child. Courts have considered a number of factors in determining a child's best interests, including:

- The seriousness of the harm the child is suffering or the substantial likelihood that the child will suffer serious harm without treatment

- The risks to the child's life or health inherent in the proposed treatment

- The risks to the child's life or health inherent in alternatives to the proposed treatment, including no treatment
- The child's age
- Any preferences the child has expressed[14]

In cases in which the child is likely to die without treatment, courts have uniformly authorized treatment for the child. In *In the Matter of Elisha McCauley*,[15] the court authorized the medical staff of a hospital to provide an eight-year old girl with "all reasonable medical care which in their judgment is necessary to preserve the patient's life and health, including but not limited to the administration of blood and/or blood products, throughout the entire course of her treatment for leukemia and related conditions." The court based its order on the judge's findings that, while the chances of the child's leukemia being brought into remission with blood transfusions and chemotherapy were "unspecified," without treatment the child faced "certain death."

The courts are not as likely to issue such an order, however, if the child is closer to majority and consequently has greater rights to the free exercise of religion and to refuse even life-sustaining treatment. *In re E.G.* involved similar facts to *McCauley*, but the "child" was 17 years old. In reversing a lower court's order authorizing blood transfusions that had been refused on religious grounds, the state supreme court noted that the state's *parents patriae* power is strongest when the minor is immature and lacking in capacity to make decision on his or her own. It went on to note that this state power fades, however, as the minor gets older and disappears upon reaching adulthood.[16]

Courts have even authorized medical treatment for a child over parental objection when the child's life was not in imminent danger. In *Mitchell v. Davis*,[17] the court awarded custody of a 12-year old boy to a juvenile officer for the purpose of obtaining medical treatment for the child's swollen leg, which was caused by arthritis or complications from rheumatic fever. The child had lost considerable weight and was in pain, but there was no immediate threat to his life.

Other courts have authorized operations to correct a physical deformity,[18] to remove a child's adenoids and tonsils,[19] and continued treatment of a three-year old boy who no longer showed signs of cancer to ensure the disease would not recur.[20] The reasoning of the courts is that the state should not have to hold its protective power in abeyance until potential harm is actual. The purpose of such court orders is to prevent risk, not to ignore it.[21]

Thus, courts may authorize medical treatment of minors despite their parents' refusal to consent to the treatment to protect the life or health of the minors.

Incompetent patients

The issues of substituted consent for medical treatment for patients who have been rendered incompetent by illness or accident or who were never competent are more complicated than those involved in substituted consent for minors for two reasons.

First, courts have taken two different approaches in their efforts to protect incompetent patients' interests. In one approach, life-sustaining medical treatment will be continued unless clear and convincing evidence demonstrates that the incompetent person would have refused such care. In the other approach, the person authorized to give consent on the incompetent person's behalf bases the medical treatment decision on what she believes the incompetent patient would have decided if competent.

Second, courts take different factors into account in such decisions, depending on whether the patient was ever competent and, if so, whether he or she expressed any preferences regarding medical treatment or executed a document, such as a "living will" or power of attorney for health care.

The first approach to making medical treatment decisions for incompetent patients does not make any distinctions between incompetent patients who were once competent and those who were never competent. Called the objective approach, it simply requires that before life-sustaining medical treatment may be withdrawn from an incompetent patient, those seeking to withdraw it must show by clear and convincing evidence that the incompetent patient would have wanted the treatment withdrawn. Unless they make such a showing, the state's interest in preserving life is controlling, and treatment may not be withdrawn.[22]

The second approach, known as "substituted judgment," is less conservative but more complicated. Under this approach, the person authorized to consent to medical treatment on behalf of the incompetent patient tries to determine whether the incompetent person would have consented to the proposed treatment. Under this approach, an incompetent patient's family and guardian, together with the patient's doctors and the hospital's ethics committee, use their best judgment and personal knowledge of the incompetent's personal values and beliefs to determine whether the incompetent would refuse life-sustaining medical treatment under the circumstances.[23]

Some courts frown upon family decision making and require a judicial determination whether the patient would consent to the treatment if competent. Regardless of whether the decision is made primarily by a court or by the patient's family, factors usually considered in determining whether an incompetent person would consent to treatment if competent are:

- The patient's prognosis if not treated
- The patient's prognosis if treated
- The risk of adverse side effects from the proposed treatments
- The intrusiveness or severity of the proposed treatments
- The patient's ability to cooperate and assist with post-treatment therapy
- The patient's religious or moral views regarding medical care or the dying process
- The wishes of the patient's family and friends, if those wishes would influence the patient's decision

If the patient was once competent, his or her views regarding medical treatment might be gleaned from an advanced directive, such as a living will, if the patient executed one before becoming incompetent. If the patient was never competent, and was never able to form or communicate his or her views regarding medical treatment, greater emphasis is placed on the benefits and burdens of the proposed medical treatment to the particular patient to determine the patient's best interests.[24]

If a substituted decision maker determines that the incompetent patient would have exercised his or her right to refuse one treatment over the other or even to refuse lifesaving treatment, the decision maker must weigh that determination against four state interests:

- The preservation of human life
- The protection of innocent third parties
- The prevention of suicide
- The maintenance of the ethical integrity of the medical profession[25]

The most compelling state interest is its interest in preserving human life. This interest is the strongest when the person in need of medical treatment would be likely to lead a relatively normal life if treated.[28] However, the patient's right to privacy, which is the basis of the right to refuse medical treatment, becomes stronger and may overcome the state's interest in preserving the patient's life as the extent of the bodily invasion inherent in the treatment increases and the patient's prognosis dims.[27]

The state interest in protecting innocent third parties relates to the state's power to compel medical treatment against a person's wishes when that person has minor children or other dependents who may be unduly burdened emotionally or financially by the person's refusal to consent to treatment.[28] This interest, in conjunction with the interest in preserving life, may outweigh a patient's right to refuse life-sustaining treatment. One scenario in which the state's interests overcome a patient's right to privacy is when the courts compel pregnant women or women with minor children to submit to unwanted treatment to safeguard their fetuses or to prevent young children from being left motherless.[29]

The interest in preventing suicide has lost most of its force in the context of medical decision making. Courts have recognized that refusing life-sustaining medical treatment does not constitute suicide because it does not necessarily constitute a wish to die, but to allow an illness to take its natural course.[30]

The interest in maintaining the ethical integrity of the medical profession serves to ensure that healthcare providers abide by prevailing ethical practice in treating their patients.[31] Largely because of advances in medical technology, what constitutes ethical treatment of patients changes. The state's interest in maintaining the ethical integrity of the medical profession serves to ensure that the decision comports with the current view of accepted medical practice and assists practitioners in resisting unacceptable demands by families of incompetent patients.

In weighing the state interests against the patient's right to privacy, courts consider many of the same factors that were relevant in determining the patient's best interests. These decisions suggest that when a patient's condition is incurable and treatment would prove invasive and burdensome, courts are more likely to respect a decision to forego treatment; and when a patient has a reasonable chance of being cured or living a relatively healthy life if treated, courts are more likely to order even invasive, burdensome treatment.[32]

Emergency exceptions

The emergency exception to the rule of informed consent is less complicated than the exceptions for minors and incompetent patients. Essentially, under state statutes, a healthcare provider may provide medical or surgical treatment to a person without first obtaining consent when:

- In the medical judgment of the healthcare provider, treatment is reasonably necessary

- The person in need of treatment is unable to give consent and another authorized to consent on the patient's behalf is not readily available

- Delaying treatment to obtain consent would be likely to result in death or serious physical harm to the person in need of treatment[33]

Note that even when the emergency exception applies, these statutes only protect the healthcare provider from liability for unauthorized treatment, not from liability for negligent treatment. However, most states have so-called "Good Samaritan" statutes that shield persons rendering emergency aid without compensation from liability unless their treatment constitutes gross negligence or intentional misconduct.[34]

Most medical emergencies arise in one of three scenarios. In the first, a person suffers a sudden injury, and taking the time to inform the patient of the risks of treatment before providing treatment would increase the risk to life or health. For example, a healthcare provider does not have to inform a person who has been bitten by a poisonous snake about the risks of treatment before providing treatment because, "It would indeed be most unusual for a doctor, with his patient who had just been bitten by a venomous snake, to calmly sit down and first fully discuss the various available methods of treating snakebite and the possible consequences, while the venom was being pumped through the patient's body."[35]

Second, where a person suffers a sudden injury and is unable to give consent on his or her own behalf, a healthcare provider may render treatment without consent when obtaining consent from another person who is authorized to consent on the patient's behalf is not feasible. One example is provided by *Jackovach v. Yocum*.[36] The arm of a 17-year old boy had been mangled when he jumped off a train. Without waiting for the arrival of the boy's parents, the physician amputated the boy's arm to save his life. The physician was found not liable for failure to obtain informed consent.

In other cases, a patient may be receiving treatment for a nonemergency condition that suddenly worsens and requires emergency care to preserve the patient's life or health. In *Stafford v. Louisiana State University*,[37] a 64-year-old woman was admitted for treatment of ketoacidosis, a complication of diabetes, and thrombophlebitis in her left leg. Both conditions can become life threatening. The latter condition caused gangrene in the patient's leg, which deteriorated to the point where an emergency amputation of the leg was necessary to save her life. In such scenarios, as with sudden injury, there is no time to find or consult another who is authorized to give consent if that person is not present when the patient's condition changes. Such situations may also arise when a patient suffers cardiac or respiratory arrest. In fact, a healthcare provider would probably be found negligent if he or she tried to contact the patient's family to obtain consent before treating the patient.

Ideally, a healthcare provider could discuss any procedures that might become necessary during the course of the patient's treatment and obtain general consent to perform any of the specific procedures discussed if medical judgment indicates they have become necessary. However, such disclosures might not always be prudent, possible, or even helpful. A change in the patient's condition might not be foreseeable. The foreseeable needs that the patient may develop may be too numerous, and discussing every contingency would be impractical and undesirable both in terms of time and the likelihood of overwhelming the patient or family.

A healthcare provider may provide medical treatment that is beyond the scope of the patient's or substituted consent when "confronted with an emergency or an unanticipated condition and immediate action is necessary for the preservation of the life or health of the patient and it is impracticable to obtain consent to an operation which he deems to be immediately necessary."[38] However, healthcare providers should be very wary of acting beyond the scope of a patient's consent. Even if the treatment benefits the patient, is rendered with skill, and does not injure the patient, a court may hold a healthcare provider liable for battery if the patient did not consent to the treatment and the treatment was not necessary to preserve the patient's life or health. For example, in *Lipscomb v. Memorial Hospital*,[39] a physician was found liable for failure to obtain informed consent when he repaired a patient's hiatal hernia during her gall bladder surgery, even though she had refused to consent to combine the hernia surgery with the gall bladder surgery. The physician testified that, during the gall bladder surgery, he discovered that the hernia was more serious than he had thought and believed it presented a medical emergency. However, the jury apparently believed testimony that the hernia did not constitute an emergency. It found that the patient's condition did not warrant unauthorized treatment.

Conclusion

The exceptions to the general rule requiring the patient's informed consent, substituted consent, and the emergency exception do authorize physicians to provide timely medical care when the patient cannot consent. However, to ensure their proper use, the facility must provide for these exceptions in their consent policy as discussed in Chapter 8.

Notes

1. Georgia code § 31–9–2 (1991). See also Arkansas Statutes Annotated § 20–9–602 (1991); Idaho Code § 39–4303 (1991); Burns Indiana Code Annotated § 16–8–22–4 (1991); Mississippi Code Annotated § 41–41–3 (1991); Utah Code Annotated § 78–14–5 (1992).
2. See Arkansas Statutes Annotated § 20–9–604 (1991); Burns Indiana Code Annotated § 16–8–12–7 (1991).
3. Santosky v. Kramer, 455 U.S. 745 (1992); Quilloin v. Walcott, 434 U.S. 246 (1978); Prince v. Massachusetts, 321 U.S. 158 (1944).
4. Cardwell v. Bechtol, 724 S.W.2d 739 (Tenn. 1987).
5. Code of Alabama § 22–8–5 (1991); Arkansas Statutes Annotated § 20–9–602 (1991); California Civil Code § 25.6 (1992); Georgia Code Annotated § 31–9–2 (1991); Burns Indiana Code Annotated § 16–8–12–2 (1991); Mississippi Code Annotated § 41–41–3 (1991); Montana Code Annotated § 41–4–402 (1989); New Mexico Statutes Annotated § 24–10–1 (1991).
6. Code of Alabama § 22–8–4 (1991); Georgia Code Annotated § 31–9–2 (1991); Montana Code Annotated § 41–1–402 (1989).

7. Code of Alabama § 22–8–4 (1991); Montana Code § 41–1–402 (1989).
8. Burns Indiana Code Annotated § 16–8–12–2 (1991); Mississippi Code Annotated § 41–41–3 (1991); Montana Code Annotated § 41–1–402 (1989); New Mexico Statutes Annotated § 24–10–1 (1991).
9. California Civil Code § 25.7 (1992); Burns Indiana Code Annotated § 16–8–12–2 (1991).
10. Arkansas Statutes Annotated § 20–9–602 (1991); Mississippi Code Annotated § 41–41–3 (1991); Cardwell v. Bechtol, 724 S.W.2d 739 (Tenn. 1987).
11. Code of Alabama § 22–8–6 (1991); Arkansas Statutes Annotated § 20–9–602 (1991); Georgia Code Annotated § 31–9–2 (1991); Kansas Statutes Annotated § 64–2892 (1990); Mississippi Code Annotated § 41–41–3 (1991); Montana Code Annotated § 41–1–402 (1989); Utah Code Annotated § 78–14–5 (1992); Virginia Code Annotated § 54.1–2969 (1991).
12. In the Matter of Elisha McCauley, 409 Mass. 134, 565 N.E.2d 411 (1991); In re E.G., 133 Ill. 2d 98; 549 N.E.2d 322 (1989); Muhlenberg Hospital v. Patterson, 128 N.J. Super. 498, 320 A.2d 518 (1974).
13. In re Eric B., 198 Cal. App 3d 996, 235 Cal. Rptr. 22 (1987); In the Interest of D.L.E., 645 P.2d 270 (Colo. 1982); In the Matter of Hamilton, 657 S.W.2d 425 (Tenn. 1983); Mitchell v. Davis, 205 S.W.2d 812 (Tex. 1947).
14. In the Matter of Elisha McCauley, supra.
15. Id.
16. 133 Ill.2d 98, 549 N.E.2d 322 (1989).
17. 205 S.W.2d 812 (Tex. 1947).
18. In the Matter of Jensen, 54 Ore. App. 1, 633 P.2d 1302 (1981).
19. In re Karwath, 199 N.W.2d 147 (Iowa 1972).
20. In re Eric B., 189 Cal. App.3d 996, 235 Cal, Rptr. 22 (1987).
21. Id.
22. See Cruzan v. Director, Missouri Department of Health, 110 S.Ct. 2841 (1990).
23. See In re Quinlan, 70 N.J. 10, 355 A.2d 647 (1976).

24. See In the Matter of Hier, 18 Mass. App Ct. 200, 464 N.E.2d 959 (1984).
25. John F. Kennedy Memorial Hospital v. Bludworth, 452 So.2d 921 (Fla. 1984); Foody v. Manchester Memorial Hospital, 40 Conn. Supp. 127, 482 A.2d 713, 718–20 (1984).
26. Foody, supra note 25, 482 A.2d 718.
27. Quinlan, supra note 23; In the Matter of Robert Quackenbush, 156 N.J. Super. 282, 383 A.2d 785 (1978).
28. Superintendent of Belchertown State School v. Saikewicz, 373 Mass. 728, 370 N.E.2d 417 (1977).
29. Raleigh Fitkin-Paul Morgan Memorial Hospital v. Anderson, 42 N.J. 421, 201 A.2d 537, cert. denied, 377 U.S. 985 (1964) (pregnant woman compelled to have blood transfusion); In re Unborn Baby Wilson, No. 81–108 AV (Mich. Ct. App. Mar. 9, 1981) (pregnant diabetic woman compelled to have insulin administered): In re A.C., 533 A.2d 611, vacated and reh'g granted, 539 A.2d 203 (D.C. 1990), vacated and remanded, 573 A.2d 1235 (1990), aff'd, 597 A.2d 920 (1991) (terminally ill pregnant woman compelled to have cesarean section).
30. Quinlan, supra note 23; Foody, supra note 25.
31. Saikewicz, supra note 28.
32. Foody, supra note 25.
33. See Code of Alabama § 22–8–1 (1991); Arkansas Statutes Annotated § 20–9–603 (1991); Official Code of Georgia Annotated § 31–9–3 (1991); Idaho Code § 39–4303 (1991); Montana Code Annotated § 41–1–405 (1989); Nevada Revised Statutes Annotated § 41A.120 (1991); Pennsylvania Statutes Annotated § 1301.103 (1991).
34. See Bunting v. U.S., 884 F.2d 1143 (9th Cir. 1989); California Business and Professions Code § 2144, 2144.5 (1990); Connecticut General Statutes § 52–557b (1990); Florida Statutes § 768.13 (1990); Wallace v. Hall, 145 Ga. App. 610, 244 S.E.2d 129 (1978); Mississippi Code Annnotated § 73–25–37 (1991).
35. Couch v. Most, 78 N.M. 406, 410, 432 P.2d 250, 254 (1967).
36. 237 N.W. 444 (Iowa 1931).
37. 448 So.2d 852 (La. App. 1984).

38. Wheeler v. Barker, 208 P.2d 68 (Calif. 1949).
39. 733 F.2d 332 (4th Cir. 1984).

Chapter 3

When Do You Need Informed Consent?

Introduction

As a general rule, a physician must obtain his or her patient's consent, expressed or implied, to a medical procedure before performing a procedure. Obviously, however, a physician need not obtain a written consent before taking a patient's pulse. In such cases the law presumes consent. When a patient voluntarily submits to such simple procedures with apparent knowledge of those procedures, the courts will usually find implied consent. Some procedures require consent, but not necessarily informed consent. But written informed consent is necessary before performing diagnostic or therapeutic procedures on a patient. In general, practitioners should obtain consent upon admission to a healthcare facility and in certain special situations.

Treatment requiring consent

Procedures that carry no risk, such as the taking of a temperature, do not require informed consent. And, as stated above, the law presumes consent. However, because every adult patient of sound mind has a right to determine what shall be done with his or her body, a harmful or offensive touching without consent is a battery.[1] If a practitioner commits such an unauthorized touching, the patient can recover damages even if the physician was not negligent and even if the treatment benefited the patient. If the unauthorized treatment benefited the patient, damages may be minimal unless, however, the unauthorized touching was highly offensive. In such cases, a court may award punitive damages. For example, in *Lloyd v. Kull*,[2] the court awarded $500 damages for battery in a case in which the surgeon removed an insignificant mole from a female patient's thigh while she was undergoing surgery for repair of a vesicovaginal fistula even though she suffered no real harm. In *Tisdale v. Pruitt*,[3] the court awarded $5,000 in actual damages plus $25,000 in punitive damages when a doctor to whom the patient was referred for a second opinion on whether she needed a dilation and curettage (D & C) performed the operation without obtaining her consent. In cases involving significant risks, however, consent must be informed consent.

Treatment requiring informed consent

Neither the law nor accrediting institutions specify exactly what procedures require informed consent. They do, however, provide some guidance for facilities and practitioners to follow. In California, for example, a physician has a duty to disclose to his patient the potential of death or serious bodily harm if a given procedure inherently involves such known risks and if a skilled practitioner normally would provide such information under similar circumstances.[4] Louisiana's Uniform Consent Law specifies that "written consent to medical treatment means a consent in writing *to any medical or surgical procedure or course of procedures* which ... sets forth in general terms the nature and purpose of the

When Do You Need Informed Consent?

procedure or procedures, together with the known risks, if any, of death, brain damage, quadriplegia, paraplegia, the loss or loss of function of any organ or limb, of disfiguring scars associated with such procedure or procedures. . . ."[5] Obviously, any treatment posing such risks requires an informed consent under Louisiana law.

Facilities should develop a consent policy that provides for signed consent in the following cases:

- Surgery involving entry into the body
- Procedures involving more than a slight risk of harm or causing change in the patient's body structure
- Procedures involving anesthesia
- Radiological therapy
- Electroconvulsive therapy
- Experimental procedures
- Other procedures that the facility medical staff determines require informed patient consent[6]

Surgery or other procedures involving risks

Performing surgery or other procedures involving more than a slight risk of harm of causing changes in the patient's body structure obviously requires informed consent. For example, in *Canterbury v. Spence*,[7] the appellate court overturned a verdict for the defendant doctor based on the plaintiff's failure to prove negligence. Because of testimony that Doctor Spence did not reveal the risk of paralysis from the laminectomy he performed that resulted in partial paralysis and incontinence of the patient, the appellate court held that the Doctor Spence's failure to tell his patient about the nature of the risk *did* constitute negligence.

The administration of anesthesia

The administration of anesthesia also requires informed consent. In *Barth v. Rock*,[8] the court found that the jury should have been instructed that the plaintiffs did not give informed consent to the use of sodium pentothal. Both the doctor and the nurse anesthetist admitted that they had not informed the minor patient's parents of the risks of general anesthesia. Similarly, in *Brown v. Dahl and Korte and Olympic Anesthesia Services, Inc.*,[9] the appellate court found that the trial court should not have dismissed the patient's/plaintiff's informed consent claim. The plaintiff's expert witnesses testified that Doctor Dahl had violated the customary practice with regard to informed consent by his failure to apprise the plaintiff of the risks of general anesthesia and of the available alternatives and that testimony was sufficient to support the plaintiff's position.

Radiation therapy

Radiation therapy also requires informed consent. In *Nelson v. Patrick, Rombold & Kinston Radiological Associates*,[10] the appellate court upheld a jury verdict for failing to obtain informed consent to radiation therapy to reduce the risk of a recurrence of cancer. The therapy caused severe damage to her intestines. On the other hand, *King v. Bauer*,[11] upheld a verdict for the doctor/defendant because he had obtained "consent given by a patient to whom such risks incident to treatment by radiation therapy have been disclosed to the patient by a radiologist of ordinary prudence under the same or similar circumstances."

State statutes, as well as the informed consent doctrine, require practitioners to obtain informed consent to electroconvulsive therapy. For example, the Illinois Mental Health

Code[12] prohibits electroconvulsive therapy or any other hazardous services without "written and informed consent."

Experimental procedures

As to experimental procedures, informed consent to the known risks is not sufficient. *Estrada v. Jaques*[13] summarizes the informed consent requirement in experimental cases:

> [W]e hold that where the healthcare provider offers an experimental procedure or treatment to a patient, the healthcare provider has a duty, in exercising reasonable care under the circumstances, to inform the patient of the experimental nature of the proposed procedure. With experimental procedures the "most frequent risks and hazards" will remain unknown until the procedure becomes established. If the healthcare provider has a duty to inform of *known* risks for *established* procedures, common sense and the purposes of the [informed consent] statute equally require that the healthcare provider inform the patient of any *uncertainty* regarding the risks associated with *experimental* procedures. This includes the experimental nature of the procedure and the *known or projected most likely risks*.

The federal government has issued regulations requiring informed consent for experimentation involving human subjects applicable to all Department of Health and Human Services grants and contracts supporting research, development, and related activities in which human subjects are involved.[14] See Chapter 4 for a discussion of what providers must disclose in such circumstances.

Other procedures as specified by the medical staff

Obviously, these procedures are not the only ones for which the practitioner should obtain informed consent. The facility's consent policy should require the medical staff to specify other operations, tests, and procedures that require written informed consent and state that the absence from the list does not mean that the physician should not obtain informed consent. Rather, the physician should resolve any doubt about obtaining informed consent in favor of obtaining it.

Nonsurgical invasive procedures are perhaps the most difficult to decide whether informed consent is necessary. Some physicians, for example, consider informed consent for drug therapies unnecessary. A recent study showed that the invasive procedure most commonly lacking written consent was chemotherapy.[15] From a legal standpoint, considering the potential side effects of chemotherapy, obtaining informed consent would seem to be the better practice.

Special situations requiring informed consent

A number of special situations require informed consent. Such situations include:

- Retention and use of body parts
- Inoculations
- Photographs or other privacy invasions
- Blood donation and transfusion
- Religiously-motivated treatments or nontreatment
- Autopsies

- Organ donations
- AIDS testing
- Reproductive matters

Retention and use of body parts

Recently, the law has imposed a fiduciary obligation on physicians requiring them to act primarily for the benefit of the patient. For example, in *Moore v. Regents of the University of California*,[16] the Supreme Court of California required physicians seeking patients' consent to medical treatment to disclose personal interests unrelated to the patient's health, whether research or economic, that might affect their medical judgment. In *Moore*, the patient/plaintiff underwent treatment for hairy-cell leukemia at the defendant medical center. The physician obtained written consent for the removal of Moore's spleen but did not inform the patient of his intention to use the spleen for research. The doctor had Moore return for checkups during which he withdrew additional samples of blood, blood serum, bone marrow aspirate, and sperm, primarily for research purposes. Eventually, the doctor and others patented a cell line from Moore's T-lymphocytes and negotiated agreements for commercial development of the cell line and products to be derived from it without obtaining Moore's consent or compensating him.

In reversing a lower court decision for the defendant, the California Supreme Court noted that a physician who adds his own research interests to the balance between the benefits of a procedure to the patient and the risks to the patient may be tempted to order a scientifically useful procedure or test that offers marginal benefits to the patient.

The court added that the possibility that an interest other than the patient's health has affected the physician's judgment is something that a reasonable patient would want to know in deciding whether to consent to a proposed treatment. In addition, where organs or tissue excised from the patient are to be used for research, education, or transplantation, the practitioner should obtain specific consent, even though the tissue would otherwise be discarded.[17]

Inoculations

Even though an inoculation is relatively simple and straightforward and even though acquiescence may amount to implied consent, the practitioner should obtain written consent before inoculating a patient. The written consent should include the purpose of the inoculation, the nature of the substance to be administered, and any risks inherent in the inoculation.[18]

Photographs or other invasions of patient privacy

Because patients have a right to privacy and confidentiality,[19] facilities should obtain written consent to the taking of any still or motion pictures or the televising of a medical procedure, even if only for educational purposes. Further, separate consent is required for photographs or interviews by the media.[20]

Blood donations and transfusions

With the advent of AIDS, blood donations carry more risks than in the past. For example, in *Valdiviez v. United States*,[21] a patient sued for receiving blood from a member of a high-risk group for HIV. The patient/plaintiff was warned prior to transplant surgery of the risk of contracting hepatitis and syphilis from a transfusion but was not warned of the risk of AIDS. The court ruled that a reasonable person in the plaintiff's position could have declined to undergo a blood transfusion from an anonymous donor and perhaps may have even declined the surgery. Consequently, informed consent is important in both the donation and the receipt of blood and blood products.

Even though drawing blood is a low-risk procedure, the facility should obtain written consent.[22] Disclosure should include the type of tests that the facility will perform on the blood and assurance of confidentiality. Similarly, the facility should obtain informed consent to transfusions, either on a separate form or as part of the consent form to surgery. Even though the risk of contracting AIDS from HIV screened blood is remote, the consequences are so great that patients are entitled to know what could happen with a contaminated transfusion, including the remote risk of screening procedures not detecting contaminated blood.[23]

Religiously motivated treatments or nontreatment

Often a patient refuses to consent to a medically indicated treatment for religious reasons. For example, Jehovah's Witnesses have refused to consent to blood transfusions.[24] In such cases, the facility's policy should outline a procedure for requesting a judicial determination to order the treatment over the patient's objection. Depending on the particular state the facility is in, the proper procedure is to seek the appointment of a guardian to consent to the procedure or to seek a court order compelling the procedure.

The courts will appoint a guardian or compel treatment if some or all of the following factors are present:

- The patient is in need of life-saving treatment as demonstrated by expert medical evidence
- The chances of saving the patient's life are good, and the risk of death is great without the proposed treatment
- The patient's decision not to undergo the treatment is based on religious beliefs
- The patient is a primary source of support for minor dependents
- The patient is pregnant and in the last trimester of pregnancy

The court would probably refuse to intervene when:

- The patient has no minor dependents or has made ample provision for their needs
- The probability of saving the patient's life is questionable
- Other reasonable treatment alternatives exist that do not violate the patient's religious beliefs
- A state law prohibits treatment of anyone known to have religious beliefs that preclude such treatment[25]

Autopsies

In the absence of a statute requiring an autopsy, such as in cases of deaths due to violence, suicide, or suspicious or unexplained causes, or a court order for one, the facility must obtain consent to perform an autopsy from instructions left by the decedent before death or from the decedent's next of kin. The facility's policy should specify procedures for obtaining consent for autopsies.[26]

Organ donations

Organ donation certainly involves surgery and changes in the patient's body structure and thus requires informed consent as discussed above. However, because two patients are involved, informed consent requires the practitioner to communicate more information than in one-patient treatments. The physician should discuss the following issues with the donor:

- Risks and possible consequences to the donor
- Benefits to the donor, if any
- Risks and benefits to the donee
- Reasonable alternatives, if any
- Extent and scope of proposed surgery
- Length of recuperation
- Impairment of sexual function, if any, in adult donors particularly
- Extent of scarring
- Extent of work time lost or period of disability
- Follow-up care required[27]

Obviously, special rules exist when the donor is incompetent. See Chapter 2.

AIDS testing

Unless a statute provides for testing for the HIV antibody without informed consent, such as when emergency medical personnel are exposed to the blood or bodily fluids of an individual in a manner that may transmit HIV, practitioners should obtain written informed consent to HIV antibody testing over and above the consent required for routine blood tests. A positive HIV antibody test may create psychological distress, result in discrimination, and affect the availability of insurance. Without information about the nature of the test, the significance of the results, and the possible effects of a record of a positive test, a patient cannot make a reasonable decision whether to submit to the test or not. In fact, many state statutes require informed consent for HIV testing and the Centers for Disease Control guidelines for routine testing of patients require consent for testing.[28] Illinois, for example, defines "written informed consent" in HIV testing as:

> an agreement in writing executed by the subject of a test of the subject's legally authorized representative without undue inducement or any element of force, fraud, deceit, duress or other form of constraint or coercion, which entails at least the following: (1) a fair explanation of the test, including its purpose, potential uses, limitations and the meaning of its results; and (2) a fair explanation of the procedures to be followed, including the voluntary nature of the test, the right to withdraw consent to the testing process at any time, the right to anonymity to the extent provided by law with respect to participation in the test and disclosure of

test results, and the right to confidential treatment of information identifying the subject of the test and the results of the test, to the extent provided by law.[29]

This statute adds that no physician may order an HIV test without providing information about the meaning of the test results, the availability of additional confirmatory testing, if appropriate, and the availability of referral for further information and counseling.[30] Even in the absence of such a statute, practitioners should obtain informed consent to avoid liability in cases where the test could legally be administered without consent, as discussed above, especially in cases in which the results are used in a way that adversely affects the patient's interests.

Reproductive matters

Informed consent also has special requirements in reproductive matters. Some states require written consent regarding artificial insemination, especially the husband's, if a donor is involved.

In addition, physicians have a duty to disclose the risks of pregnancy, including information regarding genetically linked birth defects, the availability of tests to detect problems, the risks of such tests, and the available alternatives after a test discloses a problem.

With regard to abortion, some states have enacted legislation requiring parental consent to abortion, although such statutes may be unconstitutional. In addition, courts have found the legislation requiring graphic descriptions of the gestational age of the fetus, the possibility of pain to the fetus, and the means used to control the pain which go beyond neutral and objective medical information into the realm of religious or ethical concerns violates the United States Constitution.[31]

Conclusion

A facility can minimize litigation exposure by ensuring that its consent policy addresses the normal types of procedures requiring consent, other procedures requiring consent as determined by the medical staff, and the special situations outlined above. Chapter 4 discusses how one gets informed consent.

Notes

1. Scholendorff v. Society of New York Hospital, 105 N.E. 92 (1914).
2. 329 F.2d 168 (7th Cir. 1964).
3. 394 S.E.2d 857 (S.C. Ct App. 1990).
4. Cobbs v. Grant, 502 P.2d 1 (Cal. 1972).
5. Louisiana Revised Statutes § 40:1299.40 (1975 and Supp. 1990).
6. R. Miller, *Problems in Hospital Law*, 6th ed. (Rockville, Md.: Aspen Systems Corp. 1990), 247.
7. 464 F.2d 772 (D.C. Cir. 1972).
8. 674 P.2d 1265 (Wash. Ct. App. 1984)
9. 705 P.2d 781 (Wash. App. 1985).
10. 326 S.E.2d 45 (S.C. Ct. App. 1985).
11. 767 S.W.2d 197 (Tex. Ct. App. 1989).
12. Illinois Revised Statutes ch. 91½, ¶ 2–110 (1985).
13. 321 S.E.2d 240 (N.C. App. 1984).
14. 56 Fed. Reg. 65482 (1991).
15. Terese Hudson, "Informed Consent Problems Become More Complicated," *Hospitals* 1991 65, No. 6 (March 20, 1991), 38–40.
16. 793 P.2d 479 (Cal. 1990).

17. Arnold J. Rosoff, *Informed Consent* (Rockville, Md.: Aspen Systems Corp. 1981), 254.
18. Id.
19. See § 5.05, Current Opinions of the Council on Ethical and Judicial Affairs of the American Medical Association, 1989.
20. Arnold J. Rosoff, *Informed Consent* (Rockville, Md.: Aspen Systems Corp. 1981), 254.
21. 884 F.2d 196 (5th Cir. 1989).
22. Rosoff, *Informed Consent*, 254.
23. Fay A. Rozovsky, *Consent to Treatment*, 2d ed. (Boston, Toronto & London: Little, Brown & Co. 1991 Supp.), 53–55.
24. E.g., Application of President & Directors of Georgetown College, Inc., 331 F.2d 1000 (D.C. Cir.), rehearing denied, 331 F.2d 1010, cert. denied, 377 U.S. 978 (1964).
25. Rozovsky, *Consent to Treatment*, 423.
26. Id. 620–32.
27. Id. 580–600.
28. See, e.g., Wisconsin Statutes § 146.025 (1991); Centers for Disease Control, Recommendations for Prevention of HIV Transmission in Health-Care Settings, 36 MMWR, Supp. No. 2S, Aug. 21, 1987, 15S.
29. Illinois Revised Statutes Ch. 111½, ¶ 7303(d) (1987).
30. Id. at ¶ 7305.
31. Rozovsky, *Consent to Treatment*, 144-94.

Chapter 4

How Do You Get Informed Consent?

Introduction

Once one determines that informed consent is necessary and that the patient or another can consent, the issue becomes what the practitioner must disclose to constitute informed consent. The law looks at the answer in two respects: how much information is the physician required to disclose and by what standard should a court measure this requirement?

How much information must the physician disclose?

The law of informed consent does not require total disclosure. Rather it requires *reasonable* disclosure. A landmark informed consent case, *Natanson v. Kline*,[1] specifies the scope of a physician's duty to disclose information to obtain informed consent. The Supreme Court of Kansas held that the physician's duty to disclose extends beyond a simple disclosure of risks and requires "a reasonable disclosure to the patient of the nature and probable consequences of the suggested or recommended ... treatment, and ... a reasonable disclosure of the dangers within his knowledge which were incident to, or possible in, the treatment he proposed to administer."[2] The court required, in addition to information concerning the risks of the treatment, disclosure of the ailment, the nature of the proposed treatment, the probability of success, and possible alternative treatments. Since this case, many states have specified what the physician must disclose in statutes or administrative regulations. For example, Georgia statutes provide:

> No recovery shall be allowed against any healthcare provider upon the grounds that the healthcare treatment was rendered without the informed consent of the patient ... where:
>
> 1. The action of the healthcare provider in obtaining the consent of the patient ... was in accordance with the standards of practice among members of the same healthcare profession with similar training and experience situated in the same or similar communities; and
>
> 2. A reasonable person, from the information provided by the healthcare provider under the circumstances, would have a general understanding of the procedures or treatments and of the usual and most frequent risks and hazards inherent in the proposed procedures or treatments which are recognized and followed by other healthcare providers engaged in the same field of practice in the same or similar communities; or
>
> 3. A reasonable person, under all the surrounding circumstances, would have undergone such

treatment or procedure had he been advised by the healthcare provider in accordance with the provisions of subdivisions (1) and (2) of this subsection.[3]

What is the standard for disclosure?

The standard articulated in *Natanson*, above, is known as the *reasonable physician standard*. That case went on to note that a physician's duty to disclose is limited to those disclosures that a reasonable medical practitioner would make under the same or similar circumstances.[4] This standard is based on the view that the physician, being highly trained and experienced in complex medical matters, is in a position to know what is best for the patient. In cases following the reasonable physician standard, the patient cannot recover damages for failure to receive informed consent unless he or she can produce expert medical testimony as to what the standard practice would be in such a case and that the physician deviated from such practice.[5]

Because the reasonable physician standard made it very difficult for a plaintiff to prevail in an informed consent case, some states have adopted the *reasonable patient standard*. This standard focuses on the information needed by an average, reasonable patient rather than on what the reasonable physician would disclose. *Canterbury v. Spence* was the first case to articulate this standard:

[T]he test for determining whether a particular peril must be divulged is its materiality to the patient's decision: all risks potentially affecting the decision must be unmasked.... A risk is thus material when a reasonable person, in what the physician knows or should know to be the patient's position, would be likely to attach significance to the risk or cluster of risks in deciding whether or not to forego the proposed therapy.[6]

Thus, under the reasonable patient standard, the physician must discuss the nature of the proposed treatment, whether it is necessary or merely elective, the risks, and the available alternatives and their risks and benefits. Even a very small chance of death or serious disability may be sufficient to require discussion with the patient under this standard.[7]

Information to be disclosed

Regardless of which standard the court uses to judge the disclosure, the physician should meet either standard if he or she discloses:

- The diagnosis and diagnostic tests. This includes the medical steps preceding diagnosis, including tests, their alternatives, and the risks of foregoing a diagnostic procedure. Information about diagnostic tests should include the likely outcome of diagnostic tests, the likely benefits of diagnostic tests in determining the diagnosis, and the nature and purpose of the proposed treatment.

- The risks of the treatment. The practitioner need not disclose extremely remote risks. However, the standard for disclosure of risks varies with the degree of the probability of success and the severity of the risk. Thus, the practitioner may not need to disclose a 5 percent risk of a lengthened period of recuperation but should disclose a 1 percent risk of paralysis or an even smaller risk of death. In addition, if the practitioner knows that a remote risk would be significant to the particular patient, he or she should disclose it. The practitioner should disclose temporary discomfort, disability, or disfigurement that may result from the treatment as well as any permanent results, such as scars.

- The probable outcome of the procedure including the probability of success. This disclosure should include the likely benefits from the procedure. One case suggested that the physician should disclose both the statistical success rate for the procedure and his or her personal success rate with that procedure.

- Treatment alternatives. Physicians should disclose alternatives that are generally accepted within the medical community. These alternatives should include the alternative of foregoing the procedure, their risks, and consequences and their probability of success. An alternative treatment should not be omitted merely because it is more hazardous than the proposed treatment.[8]

Of course, you should check with your hospital counsel to determine whether your state specifies any additional disclosure requirements.

What need not be disclosed

Again, the states have two different rules as to what need not be disclosed to a patient. The majority of states, those following the reasonable physician standard, do not require physicians to reveal information regarding remote risks or those that the medical community does not recognize as being applicable to a given procedure. The states that follow the reasonable patient standard does not require the physician to disclose information that is not material or significant to the patient's treatment decision although they seldom define what is not material or significant with any particularity. Courts deciding informed consent cases under the reasonable patient standard have, however, suggested that physicians need not reveal the following:

- Risks that are known to the patient

- Risks that are so obvious that the practitioner may presume that the patient has knowledge of them

- Relatively remote risks inherent in a procedure, when it is commonly known that such risks are present but are of very low incidence

- Risks that the physician did not know about or in the exercise of ordinary care could not ascertain[9]

The therapeutic privilege

The law may excuse failure to fully inform a patient of all required information under either the reasonable physician or the reasonable patient standard if full disclosure would harm the patient. Under such circumstances, the physician has a *therapeutic privilege* to withhold information from the patient. However, courts may scrutinize any assertion of the therapeutic privilege carefully. Thus, especially in jurisdictions that use the reasonable patient standard, the physician should be sure to documents in the patient's medical records the fact that disclosure of information would have

How Do You Get Informed Consent?

harmed the patient before making the treatment decision.[10] One hospital legal manual suggests:

> To document a patient's high susceptibility to anxiety, confirmation of the doctor's observation by another medical person and/or a relative or close friend of the patient should be sought and entered on the patient's treatment record.[11]

A physician may also proceed in the absence of informed consent if the patient notifies the physician that he or she does not wish to be informed. Of course, both the (uninformed) consent and the desire not to be informed should be documented as follows:

> I, (patient's name) agree to the performance of (name of procedure). I have agreed to this procedure (list how: regardless of the risk involved, without being told information to which I am entitled, etc.) The nondisclosure of information is being done at my request and I accept the consequences of agreeing to treatment without being so informed.[12]

Emergency

A physician may provide emergency medical treatment without informed consent if the patient requires immediate treatment and is incapacitated and unable to give informed consent. Of course, the practitioner should first determine whether another can give substituted consent. See Chapter 2. The law presumes that the patient would consent in an emergency if able to do so.[13] The law defines such an emergency as a life- or health-threatening disease or injury that requires immediate treatment and, in most states, waiting for substituted consent is impossible or impractical. This doctrine also applies if, during the course of an authorized operation during which the patient is under general anesthetic, a life- or health-threatening condition arises.

The emergency exception only extends to treatment that is reasonable under the circumstances. A separate elective procedure would not be reasonable or authorized by the emergency exception. Nor should a practitioner use the emergency exception to go ahead with a treatment that the patient had previously refused before becoming incapable.[14]

Conclusion

After consulting with a healthcare attorney, your facility's consent policy should specify, in general terms, what practitioners should disclose and specify procedures for treating patients under the therapeutic privilege and the emergency exception to ensure that the situation falls within an exception and is well documented.

Notes

1. 350 P.2d 1093 (Kan. 1960).
2. Id, 1106.
3. Georgia Code Annotated § 90–21.13 (Michie 1991).
4. 350 P.2d, 1106.
5. See Richard E. Shugrue & Kathyrn Linstromberg, "Practitioner's Guide to Informed Consent," *Creighton Law Review* 24 899–901 (1990–91).
6. Id., 786–87.
7. Shugrue & Linstromberg, *Practitioner's Guide*, 905.

8. Furrow et al., *Health Law*, 338; Rozovsky, *Consent to Treatment*, 45.
9. Rozovsky, *Consent to Treatment*, 54–55.
10. Shugrue & Linstromberg, *Practitioner's Guide*, 905–7.
11. *II Hospital Law Manual* (Rockville, Md.: Aspen Systems Corp. December 1982), 52–53.
12. Rozovsky, *Consent to Treatment*, 112.
13. Shugrue & Linstromberg, *Practitioner's Guide*, 909–10.
14. Rozovsky, *Consent to Treatment*, 88–98.

Chapter 5

Liability for Failure to Obtain Consent

Introduction

A practitioner's liability to a patient harmed by failure to obtain consent differs depending on whether the plaintiff sues for battery, as in cases where the patient did not consent to the procedure at all, or sues for negligence, for failure to obtain informed consent. In addition, under some circumstances, the facility may be liable for a practitioner's failure to obtain consent or for failing to obtain informed consent.

Liability for battery

A lawsuit based on a battery—an unauthorized harmful or offensive touching—is much easier for a plaintiff to prove than one based on negligence. In battery cases, the plaintiff need not prove that the physician deviated from a professional standard of care. All the plaintiff needs to prove is an unauthorized invasion of his or her person.[1] Even if such an invasion is harmless, the battery will entitle the plaintiff to nominal (insignificant) damages. In such cases, the plaintiff may recover for all injuries caused by performing the unauthorized procedure, whether or not they resulted from negligence.

Of course, if an operation is properly performed and benefits the patient, the damages would ordinarily be minimal. However, in certain cases, the court could award damages for mental anguish resulting from the patient's belated knowledge that he or she had not consented to the procedure. And, because a battery is an intentional invasion of another's bodily integrity, the court may award punitive damages in appropriate cases.[2] For example, in *Bommareddy v. Superior Court*,[3] the appellate court upheld punitive damages in a case in which the patient only consented to tear duct surgery on her left eye, but the physician performed a cataract extraction with an intraocular lens implant on her right eye without her knowledge or consent.

A physician has few defenses to a battery. Procedural and other advantages of battery-based actions make defending such actions very difficult. The plaintiff does not have to find expert witnesses willing to testify that the physician breached the standard of care. Nor does the plaintiff have to prove a causal relationship between the physician's failure to adequately divulge information necessary for informed consent and the damage to the patient. Rather, the plaintiff only has to show that the defendant committed an unconsented-to touching. Finally, punitive damage awards are generally not available in negligence actions, but they may be awarded in battery cases even when the actual damages are minimal.[4]

Liability for failure to obtain informed consent

Lack-of-informed-consent cases are negligence actions, the same as most other medical malpractice cases. *Negligence* is

Liability for Failure to Obtain Consent

nothing more than a failure to use due care. Informed consent cases follow the general principles of negligence law. Thus, to prove that the practitioner was negligent in failing to obtain informed consent, the plaintiff must prove by a preponderance of the evidence that:

- A physician-patient relationship existed between the plaintiff and the defendant physician
- The physician had a duty to disclose certain risk information
- The physician failed to provide this information
- The physician had no justification (such as an emergency situation) for failure to provide this information
- Had the physician provided the patient with the undisclosed information, the patient would not have consented to the treatment
- The physician's failure to disclose this treatment was the proximate cause of the plaintiff's injury and the damages resulting therefrom[5]

Of course, what information the physician must disclose is judged by either the reasonable physician standard or the reasonable patient standard as explained in Chapter 4. If the state is a reasonable physician standard jurisdiction, the plaintiff must prove that the physician failed to disclose information that reasonable practitioners would divulge under like circumstances.

A violation of reasonable patient standard is easier for the patient/plaintiff to prove. In such cases, the plaintiff must prove that the physician failed to disclose what a reasonable patient would want to know or need to know in order to make the decision.[6] This standard is more difficult for the physician to defend against because expert testimony supporting the physician/defendant can be discounted. The jury could find that a doctor acted unreasonably in failing to disclose certain information even when unrebutted expert medical testimony states that good medical practice would not require the disclosure of such information. In other words, the standard is the reasonable patient's perception and, in court, a jury's perception of that perception.

Regardless of which standard of disclosure applies, the plaintiff has a greater burden of showing causation—a cause-and-effect relationship between the physician's failure to adequately disclose risk information and damage to the patient—in a negligence action than in a battery action. This relationship only exists when the plaintiff proves that disclosure of the risk inherent in a treatment would have resulted in the plaintiff deciding against the treatment.

The courts measure whether the patient/plaintiff would have foregone the treatment using one of two tests: the subjective test and the objective test. The subjective test focuses on the patient, and he or she may satisfy it simply by testifying that disclosure of the risk would have resulting in declining the treatment. This standard is obviously very favorable to the patient. Thus, most courts follow the objective test—whether a prudent person in the patient's position would have declined the treatment if properly informed of all risks.

The issue of damages is also more complex in lack of informed consent cases than in battery cases. Generally, the measure of damages is the risk that materializes—the difference between the plaintiff's condition without having the treatment and the plaintiff's condition after having the treatment. However, many courts apply the so-called *benefits doctrine*, under which complications of surgery that were not disclosed are offset by benefits received from the surgery. In such cases, if the jury finds that the practitioner breached the standard of disclosure, the judge instructs the jury to subtract the benefits received from the procedure from the damages caused by the procedure.[7]

Facility liability for a practitioner's failure to obtain consent

One of the major themes of healthcare law in the last half century as been the erosion of the doctrine that exempted hospitals from the general rule that corporations are responsible for the acts of their employees. As charities, hospitals were generally immune from liability until the 1950s. Since then, however, the courts have greatly expanded hospital liability, largely in recognition of the increasing importance of hospitals in providing healthcare and supervising their staffs.[8]

Broadly speaking, a hospital is liable for the negligence or other torts committed by its employees and is not liable for those acts committed by independent contractors unless one of the following conditions exists:

- The facility exercises such a high degree of control over the independent contractor practitioner that the law will find an employee relationship.

- The facility holds itself out as providing services to patients through a practitioner, even though the practitioner is an independent contractor. For example, in *Hardy v. Brantley*,[9] the court found the facility liable for the negligence of an independent contractor because the plaintiff sought emergency care from the hospital even though he had never heard of the physician. The court found that in such circumstances, the hospital is responsible for the negligence. For example, in *Beeck v. Tucson General Hospital*,[10] the fact that the hospital had the right to control the standards of performance of an independent contractor radiologist created an employee-employer relationship so that the hospital could be liable for the radiologist's negligence.

- The law finds that the facility has a duty that it may not delegate to an independent contractor. In *Jackson v. Power*,[11] the court found that the hospital had a nondelegatable duty to provide nonnegligent physician emergency room care. The hospital was compelled to comply with state regulations requiring a physician in the emergency room at all times and had to comply with Joint Commission on the Accreditation of Hospitals (now Healthcare Organizations) standards requiring assurance of the quality control of the emergency room. Under these circumstances, the court reasoned, the hospital could not delegate these activities and could be liable for the torts of independent contractor emergency room physicians.

All healthcare institutions are liable for negligence in maintaining their facilities; for providing and maintaining medical equipment; for hiring, supervising and retaining staff, and for failing to have procedures in place to protect patients.[12] The leading case, *Darling v. Charleston Community Memorial Hospital*,[13] found the hospital directly liable for failure of the staff and administration to properly monitor and supervise the delivery of healthcare within the hospital.

Thus, a facility could be liable for a battery if a physician-employee performed an unauthorized procedure or if an independent contractor did so when the facility is held liable for the acts of independent contractors. Similarly, the facility could be held liable for negligence in cases involving failure to obtain informed consent if it did not properly monitor and supervise the obtaining of informed consent.

In *Magana v. Elie*,[14] the court reversed a decision in favor of the defendant hospital finding that a jury should determine whether the hospital had a duty to require physicians to whom it grants use of its facilities to advise patients of the risks inherent in treatment rendered within the facilities. The court noted that if the standard of care requires hospitals to take affirmative steps to require the physician to advise his or her patients of the risks of medical procedures, a failure to do so could be negligence. Note that the Joint Commission on Accreditation of Healthcare Organizations specifies that patients have the right to complete and current information concerning diagnosis, treatment, and any known prognosis, the right to reasonably informed participation in decisions involving health care, and the right to refuse treatment to the extent permitted by law.[15]

Conclusion

Liability for failure to obtain informed consent can be very costly. For example, one patient received a $500,000 jury award after he received a blood transfusion without his parent's permission.[16] Yet a practitioner can avoid this type of liability more easily than other types of malpractice. The remaining chapters will assist you to do so by detailing state and federal laws on informed consent, discussing facility consent policies, and how to actually go about obtaining informed consent.

Notes

1. Restatement (Second) of Torts sec. 13 (1965) specifies that a person is subject to liability to another for battery if:

    a. he acts intending to cause a harmful or offensive contract with the person of the other or a third person, or an imminent apprehension of such a contact, and

    b. a harmful contact with the person of the other directly or indirectly results.

2. Perna v. Pirozzi, 457 A.2d 431 (N.J. 1983).
3. 222 Cal. App. 3d 1017, 272 Cal. Rptr. 246 (1990).
4. Furrow et al., *Health Law*, 326–27.
5. Rozovsky, *Consent to Treatment*, 60.
6. Id., 61–2.
7. See, e.g., Gracis v. Meiselman, 531 A.2d 1373 (N.J. Super. 1987).
8. Furrow et al., *Health Law*, 222.
9. 471 So.2d 358 (Miss. 1985).
10. 500 P.2d 1153 (Ariz. 1972).
11. 743 P.2d 1376 (Alaska 1987).
12. Furrow et al., *Health Law*, 239.
13. 211 N.E. 253 (Ill. 1965), certiorari denied 383 U.S., 946 (1966).
14. 439 N.E.2d 1319 (Ill. App. 1982).
15. Joint Commission on Accreditation of Healthcare Organizations, *Accreditation Manual for Hospitals*, 1991 xiii (1990).
16. Terese Hudson, "Informed Consent Problems Become More Complicated," *Hospitals* 1991 65(6), 38–40 (1991).

Chapter 6

Federal Informed Consent Laws

Introduction

The Federal Tort Claims Act (FTCA)[1] makes the United States liable for the wrongful act or omission of any employee of the government while acting within the scope of his or her employment. Because no federal common law of negligence exists, courts determine whether a federal employee was negligent by applying the law of the state that the negligent act occurred in. Thus, state law governs informed consent issues in federal hospitals.[2]

Although the federal government does not have an overall informed consent law, it has specified informed consent requirements in specific areas, most notably for experimentation involving human subjects. These regulations provide a mechanism of institutional review when human subjects are involved in research and set the requirements for informed consent that must be obtained from all subjects.[3]

Informed consent for research

Both the Department of Health and Human Services (HHS) and the Food and Drug Administration (FDA) have informed consent regulations governing research.[4] The elements of the informed consent guidelines are as follows:

Basic elements of informed consent

In seeking informed consent, the following basic information shall be provided to each subject:

- A statement that the study involves research, an explanation of the purposes of the research, the expected duration of the subject's participation, a description of the procedures to be followed, and identification of any experimental procedures

- A description of any reasonably foreseeable risks or discomforts to the subject

- A description of any benefits to the subject or others benefits that might reasonably be expected from the research

- A disclosure of appropriate alternative procedures or courses of treatment, if any, that might be advantageous to the subject

- A statement that describes the extent, if any, to which confidentiality of records identifying the subject will be maintained and notes the possibility that the FDA may inspect the records

- For research involving more than minimal risk, an explanation as to whether any compensation and any medical treatments are available if injury occurs and, if so, what they consist of or where further information may be obtained

- An explanation of whom to contact for answers to pertinent questions about the research and research subject's rights and whom to contact in the event of research-related injury to the subject

- A statement that participation is voluntary, that refusal to participate will involve no penalty or loss of benefits to which the subject is otherwise entitled, and that the subject may discontinue participation at any time without penalty or loss of benefits to which the subject is otherwise entitled

Additional elements of informed consent

When appropriate, one or more of the following elements of information shall also be provided to each subject:

- A statement that the particular treatment or procedure may involve risks to the subject (or the embryo or fetus, if the subject is or may become pregnant) that are currently unforeseeable

- Anticipated circumstances under which the subject's participation may be terminated by the investigator without regard to the subject's consent

- Any costs to the subject that may result from participation in the research

- The consequences of a subject's decision to withdraw from the research and procedures for orderly termination of participation by the subject

- A statement that significant new findings developed during the course of the research may relate to the subject's willingness to continue participation will be provided to the subject

- The anticipated number of subjects involved in the study

These guidelines add that their requirements are not intended to preempt any applicable federal, state, or local laws which require the disclosure of additional information for informed consent to be effective and that the requirements do not limit the authority of a physician to provide emergency medical care to the extent applicable laws permit.[5]

Applicability of informed consent requirements

These informed consent requirements are applicable to all HHS grants and contracts supporting research, development, and related activities in which human subjects are involved. Institutions which receive HHS research support are bound to follow these regulations in all their research whether HHS directly funds the research or not.[6]

The primary difference between the FDA rules and the HHS rules is in exceptions and waivers. HHS permits alteration of consent only under certain situations, such as where the research involves no more than minimal risk and could not practically be conducted without alteration of consent requirements. The FDA permits such alteration when the subject's life is in danger, particularly in the use of experimental drugs. To alter consent procedures, all of the following must be true:

- The human subject is confronted by a life-threatening situation necessitating the use of the test article

- Informed consent cannot be obtained from the subject because of an inability to communicate with, or obtain legally effect consent from, the subject

- Time is not sufficient to obtain consent from the subject's legal representative

- An alternative method of approved or generally recognized therapy that provides an equal or greater likelihood of saving the life of the subject is not available[7]

HHS regulations require each institution to have an Institutional Review Board (IRB). Each IRB must consist of five members with varying backgrounds to promote complete and adequate review of research activities and to have the competence to evaluate the acceptability of the proposed research.[8] The function of an IRB is to review all research proposals that involve an institution's patients to determine whether they will be placed at risk and, if so, whether:

- The risks to the subject are outweighed by the sum of the benefit to the subject and the importance of the knowledge to be gained as to warrant a decision to allow the subject to accept these risks

- The rights and welfare of any such subjects will be adequately protected

- Legally effective informed consent will be obtained by adequate and appropriate methods[9]

Other federal guidance

Healthcare providers not involved in research need not observe the above requirements. Nor does involvement with the Medicare or Medicaid programs mandate observance of those requirements. However, under section 1865 of the Social Security Act,[10] a facility meets Medicare's Conditions of Participation if it is accredited by the Joint Commission on Accreditation of Healthcare Organizations. *The Accreditation Manual for Hospitals, 1991* specifies that patients have the right to complete and current information concerning diagnosis, treatment, and any known prognosis, the right to reasonably informed participation in decisions involving health care, and the right to refuse treatment to the extent permitted by law.[11]

In addition, the Omnibus Budget Reconciliation Act (OBRA) enacted protections for residents of nursing homes. It provides nursing home residents the right to be fully informed in advance about care and treatment, to be fully informed in advance of any changes in care or treatment that may affect the resident's well being, and (except with respect to an incompetent resident) to participate in planning care and treatment or changes in care and treatment.[12]

Conclusion

Thus, if your facility conducts research, is certified for federal funds, or is a nursing home, you should follow the federal guidelines discussed in this chapter in addition to any state laws governing informed consent. For such state laws, turn to the next chapter.

Notes

1. 28 U.S.C. § 1346(B) (1992).
2. See, e.g., Harrigan v. United States, 408 F. Supp 177 (E.D. Pa 1976); Roll v. United States, 548 F. Supp. 97 (E.D. Mo. 1982).
3. Department of Health, Education and Welfare, *The Institutional Guide to DHEW Policy on Protection of Human Subjects*, DHEW Publication No. 72–102 (Washington D.C.: U.S. Government Printing Office No. 1740–0326, December 1970); 45 C.F.R. Part 46. See generally, Arnold J. Rosoff, *Informed Consent: A Guide for Health Care Providers* (Rockville, Md.: Aspen Systems Corp. 1981), 261 (hereinafter *Guide for Health Care Providers*).

4. The general requirements for HHS are in 45 C.F. R. Part 46 and for FDA are in 21 C.F.R. parts 50, 71, 171, 180, 310, 312, 314, 320, 330, 361, 430, 431, 601, 630, 812, 813, 1003, and 1010.
5. 56 Fed. Reg. 65482 (1991).
6. Rosoff, *Guide for Health Care Providers*, 261.
7. Dennis Moloney, Protection of Human Research Subjects: A Practical Guide to Federal Laws and Regulations (New York: Plenum Press, 1984), 140.
8. 21 C.F.R. Parts 50 and 56, 56 Fed. Reg. 28025, § 56.107 (a) (1991).
9. 45 C.F. R. § 46.102 (b) (1991).
10. 42 U.S.C. §§ 1395x(e), 1395bb (1992).
11. Joint Commission on Accreditation of Healthcare Organizations, *Accreditation Manual for Hospitals*, 1991 xiii (1990).
12. 42 U.S.C. §§ 1395i–3(h) & 1396r(h) (1992).

Chapter 7

State Informed Consent Laws

Introduction

State informed consent laws vary widely. Some states have enacted comprehensive informed consent statutes. Others have only enacted statutes governing informed consent for particular procedures, such as AIDS testing. Still others rely on judicial decisions to specify the requirements for informed consent.

Alabama

Alabama has a statute specifying the degree of care required. It specifies that, in performing professional services for a patient, the practitioner's duty to the patient shall be to exercise such reasonable care, diligence, and skill as similar practitioners in the same general neighborhood and in the same general line of practice, ordinarily have and exercise in a like case. In the case of a hospital rendering services to a patient, the hospital must use that degree of care, skill and diligence used by hospitals generally in the community.[1]

In interpreting this statute, the Alabama Supreme Court has held that it adopts the traditional view that the doctor's duty to obtain the informed consent of his patient must be measured by a professional medical standard.[2] Alabama law also requires informed consent for HIV testing.[3]

Alaska

Alaska statutes specify that a healthcare provider is liable for failure to obtain the informed consent of a patient if the patient establishes by a preponderance of the evidence that the provider has failed to inform the patient of the common risks and reasonable alternatives to the proposed treatment or procedure and that, if the patient had had that information, he would not have consented to the proposed treatment or procedure. The statute adds that healthcare provider is not liable for medical malpractice based upon an alleged failure to obtain informed consent if:

- The risk not disclosed is too commonly known or is too remote to require disclosure

- The patient stated to the healthcare provider that she would undergo the treatment or procedure regardless of the risk involved or that she did not want to be informed of the matters to which she would be entitled to be informed

- Under the circumstances, consent by or on behalf of the patient was not possible

- The healthcare provider, after considering all of the attendant facts and circumstances, used reasonable discretion regarding the manner and extent that the alternatives or risks were disclosed to the patient. Under these circumstances, the healthcare provider reasonably believed that a full disclosure would have a substantially adverse effect on the patient's condition[4]

Arizona

Arizona statutes prohibit medical malpractice actions based on an assault and battery theory.[5]

Arizona requires written informed consent for HIV testing with certain exceptions.[6]

Arizona courts specify that the duty of disclosure of the risks of a medical procedure is measured by the usual practices of the medical profession.[7]

Arkansas

Arkansas statutes provide that where the patient/plaintiff claims that a medical care provider failed to supply adequate information to obtain the informed consent of the injured person, the patient/plaintiff has the burden of proving that the treatment was performed in other than an emergency and that the provider did not supply that type of information customarily given a patient by other providers with similar training and experience in a locality similar to that in which the provider practices. The statute notes that the following are material issues:

- Whether a person of ordinary intelligence and awareness in a position similar to that of the injured person could reasonably be expected to know of the risks inherent in the treatment
- Whether the injured person knew of such risks
- Whether the injured person would have undergone the treatment regardless of the risk or whether he or she did not wish to be informed of the risk

- Whether it was reasonable for the medical care provider to limit disclosure of information because such disclosure would adversely and substantially affect the injured person's condition[8]

Another statute provides for exceptions when informed consent is unnecessary for HIV testing.[9]

California

California has a number of statutes pertaining to informed consent. One exempts a physician from liability for damages for failure to obtain informed consent if:

- The patient was unconscious

- The procedure was undertaken without consent because the physician reasonably believed it should be undertaken immediately and insufficient time existed to fully inform the patient

- The patient was legally incapable of giving consent and the physician reasonably believed it should be undertaken immediately and insufficient time existed to obtain substituted consent[10]

Another statute requires standard written consent forms for treatment of persons involuntarily detained.[11] The Civil Code provides procedures for consent to the care of minors.[12]

Colorado

Colorado law specifies that hospitals and other facilities having in excess of 50 beds must post a policy statement specifying, among other concerns, "a clarification of a physician's duty to provide informed consent."[13] Another statute requires written informed consent for electroconvulsive treatment.[14] Colorado also specifies the ability of an agent to consent to medical treatment under a durable power of attorney.[15]

Connecticut

Connecticut statutes require informed consent for treatment of patients under the direction of the commissioner of mental retardation[16] and for HIV testing.[17]

Connecticut courts specify that, in order to obtain a patient's informed consent, a physician's disclosure should include:

- The nature of the procedure
- The risks and hazards of the procedure
- The alternatives to the procedure
- The anticipated benefits of the procedure[18]

The physician must provide the patient with the information that a reasonable patient would have found material for making a decision whether to consent to a course of therapy.[19]

Delaware

Delaware defines *informed consent* as "the consent of a patient to the performance of healthcare services by a health care provider given after the healthcare provider has informed the patient, to an extent reasonably comprehensible to general lay understanding, of the nature of the proposed procedure or treatment and of the risks and alternatives to treatment or diagnosis which a reasonable patient would consider material to the decision whether or not to undergo the treatment or diagnosis."[20] A patient may not recover damages based on a lack of informed consent unless:

- The injury involved an nonemergency treatment
- He or she proves by a preponderance of the evidence that the provider did not supply information regarding such treatment to the extent customarily given to patients by other providers with similar training and experience in the same or similar communities

The following are defenses to a suit based on lack of informed consent:

- A person of ordinary intelligence and awareness in a similar position could reasonably be expected to appreciate and comprehend hazards inherent in the treatment
- The injured party assured the provider he or she would undergo the treatment regardless of the risk involved or that he or she did not want to be given the information
- The provider reasonably limited the extent of disclosure of the risks because further disclosure would adversely and substantially affect the injured party's condition[21]

Delaware also requires written informed consent for pharmaceutical research[22] and for HIV testing.[23]

Florida

The Florida Medical Consent Law provides that the medical practitioner is not liable for treating, examining, or operating on a patient without his or her informed consent when:

- The action of the practitioner in obtaining the consent was in accordance with the accepted standard of medical practice among members of the medical profession with similar training and experience in the same or similar medical community; and

- A reasonable person, from the information provided by the practitioner, under the circumstances, would have a general understanding of the procedure, the medically acceptable alternatives, and the substantial risks or hazards inherent in the proposed treatment which are recognized by other practitioners in the same or similar community who perform similar treatments; or

- The patient would reasonably, under all the circumstances, have undergone such treatment had he been advised as above.

Under this statute, a written consent with the information above is presumed valid unless it was obtained by the fraudulent misrepresentation of a material fact.[24]

Florida statutes also require written informed consent for HIV testing,[25] for treatment in mental health facilities,[26] and provides for healthcare surrogates to consent for those who become incompetent.[27]

Georgia

Georgia law provides that a written consent to treatment that discloses in general terms the treatment or course of treatment in connection with which it is given and is signed by the patient or other person authorized to consent for the patient is conclusively presumed to be valid unless it was obtained fraudulently.[28] However, if no written consent exists, the patient may recover in an action for battery.[29]

Hawaii

The Hawaii Code requires the Board of Medical Examiners to establish informed consent standards, including provisions designed to reasonably inform a patient or a patient's guardian of:

- The condition being treated
- The nature and character of the proposed treatment or surgical procedure
- The anticipated results
- The recognized alternative forms of treatment
- The recognized serious possible risks, complications, and anticipated benefits involved in the treatment or surgical procedure, and in the recognized possible alternative forms of treatment, including nontreatment[30]

Hawaii also requires informed consent for HIV testing or disclosure[31] and for any nonemergency treatment for mental illness.[32]

Idaho

Idaho provides that consent for treatment is valid if the person giving it is sufficiently aware of pertinent facts regarding the need for, the nature of, and the significant risks ordinarily attendant upon such care, that permit the giving or withholding of consent to be a reasonably informed decision. The law deems any such consent to be valid if the practitioner has made such disclosures and given such advice as would ordinarily be made and given under the same or similar circumstances by a similar practitioner in the same community.[33] A written consent is presumptively valid in the absence of convincing proof that it was secured by fraud.[34]

Illinois

Illinois requires written consent by nursing home patients for experimental medical research or treatment,[35] and for HIV testing under certain circumstances.[36] In general, Illinois requires the physician to provide such information to the patient as a reasonable practitioner would disclose in the same or similar circumstances.[37]

As to developmentally disabled children, facilities must provide information, referral, and counseling services to ensure informed consent by the parents.[38]

Indiana

Indiana statutes specify that if a patient's written consent is signed by the patient or the patient's authorized representative, is witnessed by a person at least 18 years old, and is explained orally or in writing before a treatment is undertaken, it is assumed to be an informed consent. Such consent must include:

- The general nature of the patient's condition
- The proposed treatment, procedure, examination, or test
- The expected outcome of the treatment, procedure, examination, or test
- The material risks of the treatment, procedure, examination, or test

- The reasonable alternatives to the treatment, procedure, examination, or test[39]

Indiana also requires informed consent to blood testing for HIV.[40]

Iowa

In Iowa, the patient's right to make an informed decision about submitting to a particular medical procedure requires the doctor to disclose all material risks involved in the procedure. The doctor's duty is shaped by the patient's need for information sufficient to make a truly informed and intelligent decision, rather than what the medical community would deem material.[41]

Kansas

Kansas law makes using experimental forms of therapy without proper informed consent unprofessional conduct.[42] A physician must inform the patient of the nature and probable consequences of the suggested or recommended treatment, including possible dangers within his or her knowledge if a physician would disclose them under the same or similar circumstances.[43]

Kentucky

In Kentucky, a person who signs a general consent form for the performance of medical procedures and tests, is not required to also sign or be presented with a specific consent form relating to tests to determine HIV infection. However, a general consent form shall instruct the patient that as part of the medical procedures or tests, the patient may be tested for HIV infection, hepatitis, or any other blood-borne infectious disease if the doctor orders the test for diagnostic purposes.[44]

The law deems a patient to have given informed consent where:

- The action of the provider in obtaining consent was in accordance with the accepted standard of medical practice among members of the profession with similar training and experience; and

- A reasonable individual, from the information provided by the provider under the circumstances, would have a general understanding of the procedure and acceptable alternative procedures and substantial risks inherent in the proposed treatment which are recognized among other providers who perform similar treatments.[45]

Louisiana

Written consent to medical treatment means a consent in writing that (a) sets forth in general terms the nature and purpose of the procedure, together with the known risks, if any, of death, brain damage, quadriplegia, paraplegia, the loss or loss of function of any organ or limb, of disfiguring scars associated with such procedure; (2) acknowledges that such disclosure of information has been made and that all questions about the procedure have been answered in a satisfactory manner; and (c) is signed by the patient or person with legal authority to consent on behalf of the patient.

Such consent is presumed to be valid in the absence of proof that the consent was induced by misrepresentation of material facts. The only ground for recovery for failure to adequately disclose risks is that of negligence in failing to disclose the risks that could have influenced a reasonable person in making a decision to give or withhold consent.[47] Louisiana also requires written informed consent for HIV testing.[47]

Maine

Maine law limits liability for lack of informed consent. A healthcare provider is not liable for giving treatment without the informed consent of the patient or one authorized to consent for the patient when:

- The action of the practitioner in obtaining the consent was in accordance with the standards of practice among members of the same healthcare profession with similar training and experience in the same or similar communities

- A reasonable person, from the information provided by the practitioner, would have a general understanding of the treatments and of the usual and most frequent risks inherent in the proposed treatments which are recognized by other practitioners in the same field in the same or similar communities

- A reasonable person, under all surrounding circumstances, would have undergone such treatment had that person been advised as above

Under this statute, a written, signed consent is presumed to be valid unless the plaintiff proves it was obtained through fraud, deception, or misrepresentation of material fact.[48]

Maine also specifies that informed consent for HIV testing is consent that is based on an actual understanding by the person to be tested and is wholly voluntary and free from express or implied coercion.[49] The understanding of the person to be tested must have the following characteristics:

- That the test is being performed
- The nature of the test
- The persons to whom the results of that test may be disclosed
- The purposes for which the test results may be used
- Any reasonably foreseeable risks and benefits resulting from the test

Maryland

Maryland statutes specify that consent to HIV testing must be on a uniform written HIV informed consent form that is separate and distinct from all other forms.[50] Maryland also provides that nursing homes must have the informed consent of residents before the resident participates in experimental research.[51]

Maryland courts specify that the duty to disclose for informed consent requires the physician to reveal the nature of the ailment, the nature of the proposed treatment, the probability of success of the contemplated therapy and its alternatives, and the risk of unfortunate consequences associated with such treatment. The scope of these communications is measured by the patient's need and that need is whatever is material to the patient's decision.[52]

Massachusetts

Hospital patients have the right to informed consent to the extent provided by law.[53]

The standard of informed consent derives from the standard of care and skill of the average member of the profession practicing the specialty, taking into account the advances in the profession.[54] If the practitioner departs from that standard, the patient has not given informed consent.

Michigan

Michigan statutes require written informed consent to HIV testing that must include:

- An explanation of the test including, but not limited to, the purpose of the test, the potential uses and limitations of the test, and the meaning of test results

- An explanation of the rights of the test subject including, but not limited to:

  - The right to withdraw consent to the test at any time before the administration of the test

  - The right to confidentiality of the test results

  - The right to consent to and participate in the test on an anonymous basis

  - A description of the person to whom the test results may be disclosed[55]

Michigan also specifies specific requirements for disclosure when obtaining consent for treatment of breast cancer.[56]

Minnesota

The bills of rights of residents of healthcare facilities includes the right to participate in planning treatment, including the discussion of alternatives and to refuse treatment.[57] Minnesota statutes also provide for minors to consent to certain procedures[58] and consent to HIV and hepatitis B testing.[59]

Minnesota recognizes that patients may recover for negligent nondisclosure of information if they prove:

- A duty on the part of the physician to know of a risk or alternative treatment plan

- A duty to disclose the risk or alternative program, which may be established by showing that a reasonable person in what the physician knows or should have known to be the patient's position would likely attach significance to that risk or alternative in deciding whether to consent to treatment

- Breach of that duty

- Causation—that the undisclosed risk must materialize, thereby causing harm

- Damages[60]

Mississippi

The Mississippi Code specifies who may consent to surgical or medical treatment[61] and that implied consent exists in emergencies.[62]

Mississippi courts require physicians to disclose those known risks that would be material to a prudent patient in determining whether or not to undergo the suggested treatment.[63]

Missouri

Missouri law notes that no abortion may be performed except with the informed consent of the woman upon whom the abortion is to be performed[64] and specifies requirements for informed consent for abortions performed on minors.[65] Missouri also requires informed consent for HIV testing.[66]

A Missouri court approved a jury instruction that the jury could find for the patient in a failure to inform case if the jury found that before the physician/defendant performed the surgery on the plaintiff, he failed to inform the patient about the risk of surgical wound infection, that this failure was negligent, and, as a direct result of such negligence, the patient/plaintiff suffered damage. The term *negligence* means the failure to use that degree of skill and learning ordinarily used under the same or similar circumstances by members of the physician's profession.[67]

Montana

Montana courts indicate that, in order to obtain informed consent, the practitioner must make those disclosures that a reasonable practitioner would make under similar circumstances.[68]

By statute, Montana requires informed consent for abortion,[69] for HIV testing,[70] and before a licensed direct-entry midwife accepts a patient for care.[71]

Nebraska

Nebraska statutes require and define informed consent for abortion[72] and specify that before the plaintiff may recover damages in any action based on failure to obtain informed consent, he or she must establish by a preponderance of the evidence that a reasonably prudent person in the patient's/plaintiff's position would not have undergone the treatment if properly informed and that the lack of informed consent was the cause of the injury and its damages.[73]

Nevada

In Nevada, the law conclusively presumes consent when the physician has done the following:

- Explained to the patient, in general terms without specific details, the procedure to be undertaken

- Explained to the patient alternative methods of treatment, if any, and their general nature

- Explained to the patient that risks may exist, together with their general nature and extent, without enumerating such risks

- Obtained the signature of the patient to a statement containing an explanation of the procedure, alternative methods of treatment and risks involved as specified above[74]

Nevada statutes also detail when consent is implied,[75] that physicians may not perform abortions without informed consent,[76] and may not insert breast implants without informed consent.[77]

New Hampshire

In its statute providing for substituted consent, New Hampshire defines informed consent as occurring when a competent person, while exercising care for his or her own welfare, makes a voluntary decision about whether or not to participate in a proposed medical procedure. That voluntary decision must be based on full awareness of the relevant facts, including the medical and psychological risks and the available alternatives, the alternative of not participating in the procedure, and each alternative's attendant risks and obligations.[78] In informed consent cases, the plaintiff has the burden of proving that the treatment was performed in other than an emergency setting and that the provider did not supply that type of information regarding the treatment as would customarily have been given to a patient in the position of the injured person by other providers with similar training and experience.[79]

New Hampshire also requires informed consent for HIV testing.[80]

New Jersey

New Jersey's Bill of Rights for hospital patients notes that every patient has the right to receive from the physician information necessary to give informed consent prior to the start of any treatment and that, except for emergency situations not requiring an informed consent, shall include as a minimum the specific procedure or treatment, the medically significant risks involved, and the possible duration of incapacitation, if any, as well as an explanation of the significance of the patient's informed consent. The patient shall be advised of any medically significant alternatives for treatment, excluding experimental ones not yet accepted by the medical establishment.[81]

New Mexico

New Mexico statutes require informed consent for HIV testing, including an explanation of the test, its purpose, its potential uses and limitations, and the meaning of its results[82] and for maternal, fetal, and infant experimentation.[83]

The New Mexico Supreme Court has stated that a physician who fails to give a warning of reasonable and recognized risks inherent in a treatment after which the patient would have refused the treatment may be liable for malpractice and has adopted the objective test for causation—what a prudent person in the patient's position would have decided if suitably informed of all significant perils.[84]

New York

New York Public Health Law defines lack of informed consent as the failure of the person providing professional treatment or diagnosis to disclose to the patient reasonable alternatives and the reasonably foreseeable risks and benefits involved as a reasonable medical, dental or podiatric practitioner would have disclosed under similar circumstances. The statute limits the right to sue for lack of informed consent to nonemergency treatment, procedures, or surgery, or a diagnostic procedure involving invasion of the body or disruption of bodily integrity. The patient must prove that a reasonably prudent person in the patient's position would not have undergone the treatment if he or she had been fully informed and the lack of informed consent caused the injury.[85]

New York statutes require the use of a standardized written consent for breast cancer treatments[86] and HIV testing[87] and require human research review committees to ensure voluntary informed consent to research is obtained.[88]

North Carolina

Under North Carolina statutes, no recovery is allowed against a provider on grounds that the treatment was rendered without informed consent where:

- The action of the practitioner in obtaining the consent was in accordance with the standards of practice among members of the same healthcare profession with similar training and experience in the same or similar communities

- A reasonable person, from the information provided by the practitioner, would have a general understanding of the treatments and of the usual and most frequent risks inherent in the proposed treatments that are recognized by other practitioners in the same field in the same or similar communities

- A reasonable person, under all surrounding circumstances, would have undergone such treatment had that person been advised as above

Under this statute, a written, signed consent is presumed to be valid unless the plaintiff proves it was obtained through fraud, deception, or misrepresentation of material fact.[89]

Informed consent is required for tests for AIDS virus infection.[90] North Carolina also permits minors to consent for certain medical services.[91]

North Dakota

North Dakota laws specify who may provide informed consent on behalf of incapacitated persons[92] and require informed consent for HIV testing.[93]

North Dakota courts specify that physicians have the duty of reasonable disclosure of available choices with respect to the proposed therapy and of the material and known risks potentially involved in each.[94] The doctor must give the patient information about the nature of the procedure, the purpose it will serve, the alternatives involved, and the dangers and risks of serious complications inherent in the procedure. The doctor must make such disclosures as appear necessary to enable a reasonable person under the same or similar circumstances to intelligently consent or refuse the proposed procedure.[95]

Ohio

Ohio law presumes a written consent to be valid unless the person who obtained it was not acting in good faith, induced the consent by fraudulent misrepresentation of material facts, or that the person executing the consent could not communicate effectively if:

- The consent sets forth in general terms the nature and purpose of the procedure and what it is expected to accomplish, together with the reasonable known risks, and, except in emergencies, sets forth the names of the physicians who shall perform the intended surgical procedures

- The person making the consent acknowledges that such disclosure has been made and all questions asked have been answered in a satisfactory manner

- The consent is signed by the patient or by a person who has legal capacity to consent on behalf of the patient[96]

Ohio requires informed consent for examination for venereal disease and AIDS.[97]

Oklahoma

Oklahoma statutes require written informed consent or a substituted consent for HIV testing. If appropriate consent is provided, healthcare facilities are not liable for lack of informed consent.[98]

Oklahoma judicial opinions state that the doctor's duty to inform his or her patient of material risks and alternative treatments is judged by the patient's need to know. To recover, the patient must prove that full disclosure of the material risk or an alternative procedure would have altered the decision to consent.[99]

Oregon

To obtain the informed consent of a patient, a physician must explain the following:

- In general terms the procedure or treatment to be undertaken

- Alternative procedures or methods of treatment, if any

- Risks, if any, to the procedure or treatment

After providing this information, the physician must ask the patient if the patient wants a more detailed explanation. If so, the physician shall disclose in substantial detail the procedure, the viable alternatives, and the material risks unless to do so would be materially detrimental to the patient.[100]

Oregon statutes also require informed consent for the administration of antagonist drugs to treat drug dependency,[101] for sterilization,[102] and for treatment by experimental drugs.[103]

Pennsylvania

Informed consent is defined as the consent of a patient to the performance of healthcare services by a physician or podiatrist. The physician or podiatrist must inform the patient of the nature of the proposed procedure or treatment, the attendant risks, and alternatives to treatments or diagnoses that a reasonable patient would consider material to the decision whether or not to undergo treatment or diagnosis.[104]

Pennsylvania statutes also require informed consent to abortion,[105] to fetal experimentation,[106] and to treatment for breast disease.[107]

Rhode Island

Rhode Island has an unusual rule that considers issues of informed consent or reasonable disclosure of all known material risks as preliminary questions of fact. The judge will only submit those issues to the jury if he or she finds, after weighing the evidence and considering the credibility of the witnesses, that reasonable minds might come to different conclusions about those issues.[108]

The state also requires consent for HIV testing[109] and for human experimentation.[110]

Rhode Island courts note that, in the absence of an emergency, a physician has an obligation to make a reasonable explanation and disclosure to his or her patient of the risks of a proposed course of treatment to enable the patient to give an informed and intelligent consent.[111]

South Carolina

A South Carolina statute requires informed consent for abortions performed on minors.[112]

To prove lack of informed consent, a plaintiff must demonstrate by expert medical testimony that:

- The professional standard for disclosure in the defendant's branch of medicine; and
- The defendant's breach of that standard in the circumstances of the particular case.[113]

South Dakota

South Dakota statutes require a specific statement of informed consent to abortion[114] and for the administration of psychotropic medication to mentally ill minors.[115]

Its laws also provide that if a healthcare provider, who acts in reliance on a healthcare decision made by a person that the healthcare provider believes in good faith is authorized to make that decision, is not liable, either criminally or civilly, for that decision.[116] Substituted consent prerequisites are spelled out in another statute.[117]

The South Dakota standard for measuring performance of a physician's duty to disclose a risk is conduct that is reasonable under the circumstances. A reasonable disclosure is one that apprises the patient of all known material or significant risks inherent in a proposed medical treatment as well as the availability of any reasonable alternative treatment. A risk is material when a reasonable person, in what the physician knows or should know to be the patient's position, would be likely to attach significance to the risk.[118]

Tennessee

In a malpractice action for lack of consent, the patient must prove that the practitioner did not supply adequate information when obtaining the patient's informed consent in accordance with the recognized standard of acceptable pro-

State Informed Consent Laws

fessional practice in the community in which he or she practices and in similar communities.[119]

Tennessee statutes require consent of the parents of a minor pregnant woman[120] and of the pregnant woman herself, for an abortion.[121]

Texas

Texas law specifies that in a suit against a healthcare provider based on failure to disclose or adequately to disclose the risks involved in the treatment, the only theory under which the provider is held liable is that of negligence in failing to disclose the risks or hazards that could have influenced a reasonable person to give or withhold consent.[122]

Texas statutes also specify who may give informed consent for the immunization of a minor[123] and for consent for AIDS and related disorders testing.[124]

Utah

For a patient to recover damages for a provider's failure to obtain inform consent, the patient must prove that:

- A provider-patient relationship existed between them

- The healthcare provider rendered healthcare to the patient

- The patient suffered personal injuries arising out of the health care rendered

- The healthcare rendered carried with it a substantial and significant risk of causing the patient serious harm

- The patient was not informed of the risk
- A reasonable, prudent person in the patient's position would not have consented to the healthcare rendered after having been fully informed as to all facts relevant to the decision to give consent
- The unauthorized part of the healthcare was the proximate cause of the injuries suffered by the patient[125]

Utah law also requires informed consent or a substituted consent for blood testing when an emergency medical services provider is significantly exposed to bodily fluids[126] and for abortion.[127]

Vermont

Vermont defines lack of informed consent as the failure of the person providing professional treatment or diagnosis to disclose to the patient reasonable alternatives and the reasonably foreseeable risks and benefits involved as a reasonable medical practitioner under similar circumstances would have disclosed. This information must be provided in a manner that permits the patient to make a knowledgeable evaluation.[128]

The patient's bill of rights, another state statute, also specifies that the patient has the right to receive information necessary to give informed consent prior to the start of treatment, including, but not limited to, the specific procedure or treatment, the medically significant risks involved, and the probable duration of incapacitation as well as medically significant alternatives.[129]

Virginia

Virginia requires informed consent for abortion,[130] for testing for HIV,[131] for human research,[132] for treatment of breast tumors,[133] and for sterilization.[134]

Virginia courts have ruled that a physician owes a duty to his or her patient to make reasonable disclosure of all significant facts under the circumstances, limited, however, to those disclosures which a reasonable medical practitioner would make under the same or similar circumstances.[135]

Washington

Washington statutes specify that to win a breach of duty to secure an informed consent lawsuit, the patient/plaintiff must prove that:

- The healthcare provider failed to inform the patient of a material fact or facts relating to the treatment

- The patient consented to the treatment without being aware of or fully informed of such material fact or facts

- A reasonably prudent patient under similar circumstances would not have consented to the treatment if informed of such material fact or facts

- The treatment caused injury to the patient

This statute defines facts as material if a reasonably prudent person in the position of the patient or his representative would attach significance to it in deciding whether to submit to the proposed treatment.[136]

Residents of nursing homes have the right to give written informed consent before participating in experimental research.[137] Specific written informed consent is necessary for HIV testing.[138]

West Virginia

The West Virginia Code requires informed consent to HIV testing[139] and for laetrile use.[140]

West Virginia appellate opinions indicate that a physician has a duty to disclose information to his or her patient in order that the patient may give an informed consent to a particular procedure, such as surgery, including:

- The possibility of the surgery
- The risks involved concerning the surgery
- Alternative methods of treatment
- The risks relating to alternative methods of treatment
- The results likely to occur if the patient remains untreated

The court evaluates the disclosure based on the need of the patient material to his or her decision.[141]

Wisconsin

Wisconsin requires informed consent for HIV testing[142] and for abortions.[143]

A doctor, according to Wisconsin courts, has a duty to make such disclosures as appear reasonably necessary under the existing circumstances to enable a reasonable person under the same or similar circumstances confronting the patient at the time of the disclosure to intelligently exercise his or her right to consent or to refuse the treatment.[144]

Wyoming

The physician is required to disclose such risks that a reasonable practitioner of like training would have disclosed in the same or similar circumstances.[145]

Conclusion

Even a cursory perusal of state informed consent laws demonstrates that they vary widely. In addition, they change frequently as the legislature enacts new statutes or courts decide new informed consent cases. Make certain you consult with your legal counsel as you develop your consent policy as discussed in Chapter 8.

Notes

1. Alabama Code § 6–5–484 (1992).
2. Fain v. Smith, 479 So. 2d 1150 (Ala. 1985).
3. Alabama Code § 22–11a–51 (1992).
4. Alaska Statutes § 09.55.556 (1991).
5. Arizona Revised Statutes Annotated § 12–562 (1991).
6. Id. § 36–663.
7. Potter v. Wisner, 823 P.2d 1339 (Ariz. Ct. App. 1991).
8. Arkansas Code Annotated § 16–114–206 (1992).
9. Id. § 20–15–905.
10. California Business and Professions Code § 2397 (1992).
11. California Welfare and Institutions Code § 5326.3 (1992).
12. California Civil Code Part 1 (1992).
13. Colorado Revised Statutes § 25–1–121 (1992).
14. Id. § 13–20–402.
15. Id. § 15–14–506.
16. Connecticut General Statutes § 17a–238 (1990).
17. Id. § 19a–582.
18. Petriello v. Kalman, 576 A.2d 474 (Conn. 1990).

19. Pedersen v. Vahidy, 552 A.2d 419 (Conn. 1989).
20. Delaware Code Annotated tit. 18, § 6801 (1991).
21. Id. § 6852.
22. Delaware Code Annotated tit. 16, § 5175 (1991).
23. Id. §§ 1201 and following.
24. Florida Statutes Annotated § 786.46 (West 1991).
25. Id. § 381.0041.
26. Id. § 394.459.
27. Id. § 745.42.
28. Georgia Code Annotated § 31–9–6 (Michie 1992). See, e.g., Holbrook v. Schatten, 299 S.E.2d 128 (Ga. App. 1983); Cole v. Jordon, 288 S.E.2d 260 (Ga App. 1982).
29. Johnson v. Srivastava, 405 S.E.2d 725 (Ga. App. 1991).
30. Hawaii Revised Statutes § 671–3 (1991).
31. Id. § 325–16.
32. Id. § 334E–1.
33. Idaho Code § 39–4304 (1992).
34. Id. § 39–4305.
35. Illinois Revised Statutes Ch. 111½, ¶ 5152–104 (1991).
36. Id. ¶¶ 7304–7308.
37. Green v. Hussey, 262 N.E.2d(Ill. App. 1970).
38. Id. ¶ 2103.
39. Indiana Code Annotated § 16–9.5–1.4 (Burns 1991).
40. Id. § 16–8–7–6.
41. Doe v. Johnston, 476 N.W.2d 28 (Iowa 1990).
42. Kansas Statutes Annotated § 65–2837 (1991).
43. Wozniak v. Lipoff, 750 P.2d 971 (Kan. 1988).
44. Kentucky Revised Statutes Annotated § 214.625 (Baldwin 1991).
45. Id. § 304.40–320.
46. Louisiana Revised Statutes Annotated 40:1299.40 (West 1992).
47. Id. § 40:1300.13.
48. Maine Revised Statutes Annotated tit. 24, § 2905 (West 1991).

49. Id. tit. 5, § 19201.
50. Maryland Health–General Code Annotated § 18–336 (1991).
51. Id. § 19–344.
52. Sard et Vir v. Hardy, 379 A.2d 1014 (Md. App. 1977).
53. Massachusetts General Laws Ch. 111, § 70E (1992).
54. Johnston v. Stein, 562 N.E.2d 1365 (Mass. App. Ct. (1990).
55. Michigan Compiled Laws § 333.5133 (1991).
56. Id. § 333.17013.
57. Minnesota Statutes § 144.651 (1991).
58. Id. § 144.343.
59. See Id. § 144.762.
60. Pratt v. University of Minnesota Affiliated Hospitals, 403 N.W.2d 865 (Minn. Ct. App. 1987).
61. Mississipi Code Annotated § 41–41–3 (1991).
62. Id. § 41–41–7.
63. Barner v. Gorman, 1992 LEXIS 484 (Miss. 1992).
64. Missouri Revised Statutes § 41–41–33 (1991). The statute specifies what must be disclosed.
65. Id. § 188.028.
66. See Id. § 191.674.
67. Baltzell v. Buskird, 752 S.W.2d 902 (Mo. Ct. App. 1988).
68. Collins v. Itoh, 503 P.2d 36 (Mont. 1972).
69. Montana Code Annotated § 50–20–106 (1992).
70. Id. §§ 50–16–1003–1006.
71. Id. § 37–27–311.
72. Nebraska Revised Statutes § 28–326 (1991).
73. Id. § 44–2820.
74. Nevada Revised Statutes § 41A.100 (1991).
75. Id. § 41A.120.
76. Id. § 442.252. § 442.253 details required disclosures to obtain informed consent for abortion.
77. Id. § 449.740.
78. New Hampshire Revised Statutes Annotated § 168–B:1 (1991).

79. Id. § 507–C:2.
80. Id. § 141–F:5.
81. New Jersey Revised Statutes § 26:2H–12.8 (1991).
82. New Mexico Statutes Annotated § 24–2B–2 (1992).
83. Id. § 24–9A–2.
84. Gerety v. Demers, 589 P.2d 180 (N.M. 1978).
85. New York Public Health Law § 2805–d (Consol. 1992).
86. Id. § 2404.
87. Id. § 2786.
88. Id. § 2444.
89. North Carolina General Statutes § 90–21.13 (1991).
90. Id. § 130A–148.
91. Id. § 90.21.5.
92. North Dakota Century Code § 23–12–13 (1991).
93. Id. § 23–07.5–02.
94. Winkjer v. Herr, 277 N.W.2d 579 (N.D. 1979).
95. Wasem v. Laskowski et. al., 274 N.W.2d 219 (N.D. 1979).
96. Ohio Revised Code Annotated 2317.54 (Baldwin 1991).
97. Id. § 2907.27.
98. Oklahoma Statutes tit. 63, § 1.502.3 (1991).
99. 742 P.2d 1126 (Okla. 1987).
100. Oregon Revised Statutes § 677.097 (1991).
101. Id. § 430.545.
102. Id. § 436.225.
103. Id. § 475.325.
104. 40 Pennsylvania Statutes Annotated § 1301.103 (1990).
105. 18 Pennsylvania Consolidated Statutes § 3202 (1990).
106. Id. § 3216.
107. 35 Pennsylvania Statutes Annotated § 5642 (1990).
108. Rhode Island General Laws § 9–19–32 (1991).
109. Id. § 23–6–11.
110. Id. § 23–17.5–7.
111. Wilkinson v. Vesey, 295 A.2d 676 (R.I. 1972).

State Informed Consent Laws

112. South Carolina Code Annotated § 44–41–31 (Law.Co-op. 1990).
113. Baxley v. Rosenblum et. al., 400 S.E.2d 502 (S.C. Ct. App. 1991).
114. South Dakota Codified Laws Annotated § 34–23A–10.1 (1992).
115. Id. § 27A–15–48.
116. Id. § 34–12C–7.
117. Id. 34–12C–2.
118. Savold v. Johnson, 443 N.W.2d 656 (S.D. 1989).
119. Tennessee Code Annotated § 29–26–118 (1992).
120. Id. § 37–10–307.
121. Id. § 39–15–202.
122. Texas Revised Civil Statutes Annotated art. 4590i (West 1992).
123. Texas Family Code Annotated § 35.011 (West 1992).
124. Texas Health and Safety Code Annotated § 81.105 (1992).
125. Utah Code Annotated § 78–14–5 (1992).
126. Id. § 26–6a–2 (1992).
127. Id. § 76–7–305.
128. Vermont Statutes Annotated tit. 12, § 1909 (1991).
129. Id. tit. 18, § 1852.
130. Virginia Code Annotated § 18.2–76 (Michie 1992).
131. Id. § 32.1–37.2.
132. Id. §§ 32.1–162.16 & –162.18.
133. Id. § 54.1–2970.
134. Id. §§ 54.1–2974 & 2975.
135. Bly v. Rhoads, 222 S.E.2d 783 (Va. 1976).
136. Washington Revised Code § 7.70.050 (1991).
137. Id. § 74.42.040.
138. Id. § 69.51.040.
139. West Virginia Code § 16–3C–2 (1992).
140. Id. § 16–5A–9a.
141. Adams v. El-Bash, 338 S.E.2d 381 (W. Va. 1985).
142. Wisconsin Statutes § 146.023 (1990).

143. Id. § 146.78.
144. Peeples v. Sargent, et. al., 253 N.W.2d 459 (Wis. 1977).
145 Robal v. Bell, 778 P.2d 108 (Wyo. 1989).

Chapter 8

Facility Consent Policy

Introduction

Because of the complexity of the legal requirements of informed consent and the potential liability for failure to obtain consent, every facility should have a consent policy to ensure that practitioners obtain *and document* informed consent. Even if a practitioner has obtained a legally valid consent, he or she (or the facility if the practitioner is an employee or another basis exists for finding the facility liable, see Chapter 5) is not assured of freedom from liability unless consent can be proven in a lawsuit. If a facility has a legally sufficient consent policy, requires practitioners to follow it, and requires the use of consent forms, little likelihood exists that the facility or the individual practitioner will be found liable for failure to obtain consent.

Legally sufficient consent policy

A facility should, in connection with its healthcare attorney, develop a legally sufficient consent policy. The starting point is to locate and analyze the statutes and court decisions detailing the requirements for consent in the state that the facility is located in and determining whether any federal requirements apply. Some state statutes specify that consent obtained in compliance with them are presumptively valid. However, court decisions may not be ignored because they may modify or supplement any informed consent statutes.

The consent policy should specify:

- When consent is required. This portion of the policy should cover both procedures for determining whether implied consent exists, as in the case of emergencies, and requirements for special consent in situations that pose special risks or are required by law, such as autopsy, sterilization, human experimentation, anatomical gifts, reproductive matters, and so on.

- Who may consent, including procedures for obtaining substituted consent in cases involving minors and incompetents.

- What must be disclosed. Obviously the policy should not list risks, for example, that must be disclosed. It should, however, specify the parameters of what must be disclosed in accordance with any applicable statutes or case law.

- Who is responsible for obtaining informed consent. Normally, the attending or treating physician is ultimately responsible, but the policy may provide for designation of another physician to obtain the consent if the latter is particularly knowledgeable of the benefits and risks of the procedure and alternative procedures. Generally, a referring physician is not responsible for obtaining informed consent when a specialist performs the test or the procedure.[1] Simply stated, the person who performs the procedure should obtain informed consent to it. The duty to obtain informed consent may be delegated to a third party, such as a nurse practitioner; however, any liability for nondisclosure of material information rests with the attending or treating physician.[2]

- How consent is to be obtained, including procedures when the patient does not speak English or has other communications barriers.
- How consent is documented, including use of consent forms and documentation in medical records.

See Appendix I, sample consent policy.

Consent forms

Consent forms must be used for a number of reasons. First, many state statutes require them for certain procedures, such as HIV testing, or provide that the patient's signature on a consent form results in a presumption that the practitioner obtained a valid consent. In the absence of fraud or the misrepresentation of a material fact, the patient's signature on a general consent form should, at a minimum, absolve the practitioner from liability for a battery—an unauthorized touching. And, a detailed consent form, specifying the risks and the alternatives to a procedure, should go a long way toward mounting an effective defense to a lack-of-informed-consent claim.

Second, some state statutes or administrative regulations and the Joint Commission on Accreditation of Healthcare Organizations require documentation of informed consent in the patient's medical records.[3]

Finally, use of a good consent form can promote a dialogue between the practitioner and the patient that can lead to better results as well as reducing the likelihood of a malpractice claim.[4]

If the facility treats a large number of non-English speaking patients or patients who speak English as a second language, it may wish to have consent forms prepared in languages used by a substantial portions of its patients.[5]

Some experts break consent forms into three types: blanket consent forms, battery consent forms, and detailed consent forms.[6]

Blanket consent forms

Blanket consent forms purport to authorize the attending physician to perform any procedure he or she desires to undertake. Courts, however, have held these not to evidence consent to all procedures that may be performed in a facility because the procedures are not specified.[7] However, use of a blanket admission consent form would seem to be advisable to provide evidence of consent to routine hospital procedures, such as the taking of temperatures, etc. The blanket consent form may also obtain consent to hospital educational programs and the release of certain information, such as the patient's name, status, and so forth.

Battery consent forms

A battery form indicates that the patient or person signing on the patient's behalf has been informed of the condition he or she is suffering from, the consequences, risks, and alternatives to the proposed treatment. Such forms will protect the practitioner from a battery claim and may help to show informed consent. However, they will not automatically preclude a claim for lack of informed consent because they do not show that all material issues were discussed with the patient.

Detailed consent forms

In general, detailed consent forms, which specify not only the medical condition, procedure, and consequences, but also the risks and alternatives, are more likely to withstand judicial scrutiny and defeat a claim for lack of informed consent. However, such a form could conceivably be too detailed and exhaustive, leading to a conclusion that a risk not listed and discussed on the form was not discussed with the patient at all.

Not only should the practitioner obtain the execution of a consent form, he or she should document the disclosure and the consent in the patient's medical records. Indeed, some practitioners have taken to audio- or videotaping informed consent discussions as an additional protection against lack of informed consent suits. While going to those lengths may not be necessary, such a vivid portrayal of what the practitioner told the patient would be a powerful item of evidence for the defense.[8] Practitioners may also supplement consent forms with other materials, such as information booklets.

One expert recommends that, at a minimum, the informed consent entry in the medical records should contain:

- The description of the proposed procedure as given to the patient
- A list of the risks and benefits disclosed to the patient

- A list of any reasonable alternative forms of care, if any exist, that were disclosed to the patient
- The patient was told of others who would participate in the performance of the procedure
- The patient was told there was no guarantee of success
- When the procedure is exploratory, the patient understood and agreed to its extent and the possible removal of tissue for pathological assessment, or excision, if diseased
- The questions posed by the patient were answered
- The patient was informed of additional information that the physician considered important, such as probable discomfort, the impact on the patient's lifestyle and work, the length of recuperation, and any disability
- In the physician's estimation the patient was mentally capable of giving consent and, insofar as the physician knew, was legally competent to give consent and gave it freely
- The names of any witnesses
- The date, time, and the signature of the physician[9]

When developing a consent policy, the facility should remember that the actual process of providing information to the patient or person consenting on the patient's behalf is more important than any piece of paper documenting the consent. The form is evidence of the consent process, not a substitute for a dialogue between the practitioner and the patient.[10] One study put the use of consent forms in perspective:

- Consent forms were generally presented to the patient only after the decision was made. They rarely changed their decision because of the information in the form
- The forms were typically too complex for the average patient
- Particularly during the admission process, patients often did not read consent forms before signing them; even when they did, they seldom understood much of the material in them
- Facility staff often view consent forms as bureaucratic obstacles to be surmounted before treatment may commence[11]

Your consent policy should ensure that consent is truly informed as the result of a dialogue between the patient and the practitioner with the goal of improving medical care by involving the patient in decision making rather than merely being a bureaucratic obstacle. If it does so, it will almost certainly reduce malpractice liability as well. See Appendix II for sample consent forms.

Conclusion

By now you should be convinced that developing a legally sufficient consent policy with proper consent forms will substantially reduce potential liability for lack of consent or lack of informed consent. And such a policy can help improve patient care by making the patient a willing and informed participant in the treatment rather than just a passive object. The appendices will help you do this by illustrating a sample consent policy and sample consent forms.

Notes

1. Fay A. Rozovsky, *Consent to Treatment: A Practical Guide* (Boston & Toronto: Little, Brown & Co. 1984), 647.
2. Theodore LeBlang, & W. Eugene Basanta, *The Law of Medical Practice in Illinois* (Roschester, NY: Lawyer's Co-operative Publishing Co. 1986), 472.
3. E.g., Maryland Annotated Code art. 10, § .07.20.20 (1988); Joint Commission on Accreditation of Healthcare Organizations, Accreditation Manual for Hospitals, 1991 81, 83 (1990).
4. See Ron Winslow, "Sometimes Talk is the Best Medicine: For Physicians, Communications May Avert Suits," *Wall Street Journal* (October 5, 1989), B1.
5. Robert D. Miller, *Problems in Hospital Law*, 6th ed., (Rockville, Md.: Aspen Systems Corp. 1990), 249.
6. Richard E. Shugrue & Kathyrn Linstromberg, "Practitioner's Guide to Informed Consent," *24 Creighton Law Review* 881–82 (1990–91), citing Miller, *Problems in Hospital Law*, 247.
7. Id.
8. Id., 920–27.
9. *Consent to Treatment*, 640–41
10. *Problems*, 248.
11. Barry R. Furrow, Sandra H. Johnson, Timothy S. Jost, & Robert L. Schwartz, *Health Law, Cases, Materials and Problems*, 2d ed. (St. Paul, MN: West Publishing Co., 1991), 376–77.

Appendix I

Sample Consent Policy

CONSENT POLICY

Introduction

This policy is for use by hospital personnel, physicians, and other medical professionals. It addresses obtaining consent to treatment only (not required reports, disclosure of patient information, or other related issues) and is general in nature.

The policy and accompanying forms do not replace physician judgment and in every case physicians must use their experience and medical judgment to determine how to obtain the appropriate patient. A completed consent form is sufficient evidence of consent unless rebutted by a preponderance of evidence. The signed form does not substitute for the voluntary and informed decision of the patient or the patient's legal representative, which the physician must obtain.

Forms

All inpatients and outpatients receiving treatment at the hospital must sign a *General Consent for Treatment* form.

Hospital personnel supervise the completion of this form and place it in the medical record when each patient is admitted or receives initial treatment.

The anesthesiologist must obtain and place in the medical record a completed and signed *Consent to Anesthesia* form for all procedures in which anesthesia is used.

The physician responsible for performing the procedure must obtain and place in the medical record either a completed and signed *Consent to Operation or Procedure* form or a completed and signed *Special Consent* form before any of the following procedures are performed:

1. Surgery that involves an entry into the body, either through an incision or through a natural body opening

2. Nonsurgical procedures including administration of medicines that involve more than a slight risk of harm to the patient or that may cause a change in the patient's body structure (such as chemotherapy, hormone treatments and diagnostic procedures such as myelograms, arteriograms, and pyelograms)

3. All procedures in which anesthesia is used whether or not an entry into the body is involved (in addition to the *Anesthesia Consent* form.

4. Radiological therapy

5. Electroconvulsive therapy

6. Experimental procedures

7. Particularly invasive, irreversible or dangerous operations or procedures (such as lobotomies, sterili-

zations, abortions, and removals or refusals of life-saving treatment)

8. Procedures that may cause a change in the patient's body structure
9. Tests for the human immunodeficiency virus (HIV)
10. All other procedures for which the medical staff determines a specific explanation to the patient is required. A list of specific operations, tests, and procedures that require a consent form is attached. The absence from this list of a particular operation or procedure does not mean that the special consent need not be obtained.

Procedure

I. In general

The physician responsible for the treatment or procedure must obtain consent in a timely manner and place the appropriate signed and dated consent form in the patient's medical record. The physician should write the nature of the operation or procedure in full, without abbreviations. The physician should resolve any doubt about obtaining a consent form in favor of obtaining this evidence of consent.

Although the hospital will provide physicians with various consent forms, *it is the physician's responsibility to obtain informed consent*. A patient's consent may not be binding if the patient is under the influence of drugs or intoxicants, mental illness or other impairment of reasoning power. The test is one of medical judgment—the physician must determine that the patient has sufficient mental ability to understand the situation and to make a well-reasoned decision.

The elements the patient (or the patient's legal representative) must understand are the nature of the procedure or treatment, the possible medical risks associated with it, the benefits likely to be gained, the medical risks associated with refusal, the alternative methods of treatment, and the risks and benefits associated with such alternatives.

If the physician believes that informing a patient of these elements is medically contra-indicated, he or she should document in the patient's medical record this finding and the reasons supporting it. The physician should then obtain and document substituted consent according to the procedures described in Part II A of this policy for incompetent adults. Physicians must exercise extreme caution when relying on this type of substituted consent and should fully apprise the person who gives substituted consent. The physician should obtain a concurring professional opinion that the patient should not be advised of the facts necessary to give informed consent and document this concurrence in the medical record.

In the rare circumstance in which a physician must obtain substituted consent by telephone, another member of the hospital staff or a hospital employee should also be a party to the conversation. The physician must document the telephone consent in the patient's medical record and obtain written confirmation as soon as possible and place it in the medical record.

If an operation or procedure has not been performed within 30 days after the date the physician obtained consent, the physician must obtain a new written consent.

The person who consents to an operation or procedure may revoke consent orally or in writing any time prior to the operation or procedure. Any medical professional who is aware of revocation must immediately document it in the medical record and notify the attending physician. The operation or procedure shall not be performed until the physician has obtained a new consent.

II. Non-emergency

A. Adults (eighteen years of age or over)

The physician should obtain informed consent from a mentally competent and conscious adult.

If the adult patient is incompetent, the physician may obtain consent from the individuals listed below *after* the physician documents the following facts in the medical record:

1. The patient's guardian is unknown or cannot be located

2. The patient is unconscious, incompetent, or otherwise incapable of consenting

3. In the physician's medical judgment, the patient's medical condition, although not yet an emergency, is likely to deteriorate and should receive treatment before the adult will be capable of giving informed consent

The persons who may give substituted consent under these circumstances are as follows:

1. The judicially appointed guardian of the person

2. The persons or persons designated by the patient in a written declaration to make treatment decisions for the patient. The requirements for a written declaration appear in the hospital's *Policy for Withholding Treatment*

3. The spouse of the patient
4. An adult child of the patient or, if the patient has more than one adult child, a majority of the adult children who are reasonably available for consultation
5. The parents of the patient
6. The nearest living relative of the patient

The physician must obtain consent from the individuals in the order listed above and should rely upon consent from a lower listed class only if no individual in a prior class is available, willing, and competent to act. At least two persons should be present when the physician consults with the individual giving consent, and both witnesses should sign the consent form.

If the physician is on notice that any of the listed individuals object to the proposed treatment or procedure, he or she should allow them time to petition the court to resolve this dispute.

If the physician cannot locate the listed individuals after a thorough and reasonable search, the physician should obtain a consultation before he performs any procedure and carefully document the consultation and his efforts to locate the individuals in the medical record.

Notwithstanding the above, the physician should not proceed without a court order where any "controversial" procedure is involved as determined by the medical staff. In general, controversial procedures are those expected to produce irreversible and conceivably avoidable loss or serious limitation of important physical or psychological functions such as termination of pregnancy, sterilization, and psychosurgery.

Sample Consent Policy

B. *Minors (17 years of age or under)*

Both parents must consent to nonemergency medical treatment of a minor. If the minor's parents are separated, divorced or deceased, the legal guardian of the minor must consent. Consent for wards of the juvenile court must be given by the parents, court appointed guardian or judge, not by the foster parents.

Exceptions to this general rule include the following:

1. An unwed pregnant minor may consent to the performance of medical or surgical services relating to her pregnancy, except in the case of sterilization or abortion. A nonemergency abortion may be performed only with the consent of the parents, legal guardian, or authorization from a Circuit Court

2. An unwed minor mother may consent to the performance of medical or surgical services for her child

3. A minor may consent to medical treatment relating to his or her professed affliction with or exposure to any communicable venereal disease

4. A minor may consent to medical treatment directly related to his or her drug abuse or dependency

5. A minor who is married or has been married may consent to his or her medical treatment

6. An emancipated minor (a minor who has permanently left his or her parent's home, who has become completely self-supporting, and whose parents pay none of his or her financial obligations) may consent to his or her medical treatment

III. Emergency

The physician should follow the procedure for nonemergency situations unless delay in obtaining consent or a court order will result in the patient's death or a serious deterioration of the patient's condition. The physician should, if possible, obtain a consulting opinion before proceeding without consent. The consultation should be documented in the medical record and comply with the procedures listed below:

A. Adults (18 years or older)

The physician must sign the consent form, document the following facts, and place the consent and the documentation in the patient's medical record:

1. An emergency condition existed (delay in initiating treatment would result in the patient's death or a serious deterioration of the patient's condition)
2. The patient was not able to consent
3. Others were not available to consent for the patient

B. Minors (17 years old or younger)

The physician must sign the consent form, document the following facts and place the form and documentation in the medical record:

1. The minor was injured in an accident or suffering from an acute illness, disease, or condition
2. Delay in initiating emergency medical treatment would endanger the minor's health and immediate emergency medical care was necessary for the patient's health

3. A guardian's consent could not be obtained because:
   a. the minor was not able to reveal the identity of his guardian and such information was not known to any person who accompanied the minor to the hospital; or
   b. the guardian could not be immediately located by telephone or otherwise at his or her place of business or residence.

The physician must notify the guardian as soon as possible.

The physician should obtain the informed consent of any adult accompanying the minor, although this consent may not be valid legally and *does not* substitute for the procedures outlined above.

C. *Emergency abortions*

Where an emergency abortion is required, the physician must first obtain at least one written corroborative medical opinion attesting to the medical necessity for emergency medical procedures and to the fact that, to a reasonable degree of medical certainty, the continuation of the pregnancy would threaten the life of the pregnant woman. Such corroboration must be documented in the patient's medical record.

IV. Non-English speaking patients

When informed consent is obtained from a non-English speaking patient, a translator must assist the physician and witness the consent form. Consent forms are available in both English and Spanish. The physician should give Spanish speaking patients the form printed in Spanish. If the patient does not appear to understand either English or Spanish, the physician should give him or her the English consent form. In either case, the translator should translate the physician's explanation of the facts necessary to obtain consent in a language the patient appears to understand before the patient signs the consent form. The translator should write in this language and in English the explanation on the form. If patient comprehension is questionable, the physician should not perform the procedure until doubt about obtaining informed consent is resolved.

Appendix II

Sample Consent Forms

CONSENT FOR TREATMENT AND RELEASE OF INFORMATION BY PATIENT

Patient: _____

Attending Physician: _____

Date of Admission: _____ 19____ Time _____ am/pm
   (or treatment, if outpatient)

1. I authorize University Community Hospital ("the hospital"), its personnel, my doctor, any person under my doctor's direction or responding to his orders, and other professionals with privileges at the hospital to perform all necessary tests and procedures and to administer all necessary medications and treatments required in the course of the diagnosis and treatment of my illness.

2. I am aware that the practice of medicine and surgery is not an exact science and I acknowledge that no guarantees or representations have been made to me as a result of treatments, procedures, or examinations performed or to be performed while I am in the hospital.

3. I consent to the photographing and publication for sale or for medical, scientific, or educational purposes of any all and descriptions, photographs, or videotaping of the operations or procedures to be performed on me in the hospital. These photographs and videotapings may include portions of my body, provided the pictures and any descriptive text accompanying them do not reveal my identity.

4. I authorize the hospital to retain, preserve, use for scientific research, therapeutic or teaching purposes, or dispose of any specimens or tissues taken from my body during my hospitalization.

5. I consent to the release of medical information to other institutions or agencies accepting me for medical or institutional care, and consent to the release of medical information to my insurer.

6. I understand that my doctor and other doctors on the staff of this hospital are not employees or agents of the hospital, but are independent contractors who have been granted the privilege of using the hospital facilities for the care and treatment of their patients.

7. I impose no specific limitations or prohibitions regarding treatment other than those that follow (if none, so state):

_____.

I have read and clearly understand the above and have deleted any portions with which I do not agree. My doctor has fully explained this form to me and answered all my questions. I am satisfied that I understand the content and significance of this form.

_____   _____
Witness   Patient's Signature
                             Date: _____ Time: _____

PATIENT CONSENT TO OPERATION OR PROCEDURE

Patient: _____ Date: _____ Time: _____

1. After examining me, Dr. _____ has told me that I have_____ (name of condition or ailment).

2. My doctor has recommended _____ (name of operation or procedure). I authorize and consent to the performance upon myself of this operation or procedure by my doctor and any assistants, including hospital personnel, supervised by him who he believes are necessary and appropriate.

3. I have discussed with my doctor the following issues summarized below. My doctor has explained these issues to me, answered all my questions, and I understand that:

- A. The nature and purpose of the operation or procedure is _____.

- B. The risks and benefits of the operation or procedure are: _____.

- C. The possible or likely consequences of the procedure are: _____.

- D. The alternatives methods of treatment are: _____.

- E. The risks and benefits of these alternatives are: _____.

- F. The risks of refusing treatment entirely are: _____.

Sample Consent Forms

4. The doctor has told me and I understand that during the course of the operation or procedure, unforeseen conditions may require additional or different procedures than set forth above. I authorize and request that my doctor and his assistants perform such procedures as my doctor believes are necessary.

5. I acknowledge that no guarantee or assurance has been given by anyone as to the results or outcome of, or recovery from, these operations or procedures.

6. For the purpose of advancing medical education, I consent to the admittance of observers to the room where the operation or procedure is to be performed.

7. I hereby authorize University Community Hospital to retain, preserve, use for scientific research, therapeutic, or teaching purposes, or dispose of any specimens or tissues taken from my body during hospitalization except as specified below (if none so state):_____

_____.

8. I agree to receive blood or blood products or derivatives as deemed necessary by my doctor. I have been told and understand that a small percentage of blood recipients have an allergic or other adverse reaction to the blood they receive and that such reactions, although rare, can be serious or fatal.

9. I consent to the administration of anesthesia to be applied by or under the direction of an anesthesiologist and to the use of anesthetics he may deem desirable. I also consent to the administration of anesthesia different from that planned if it is considered necessary or advisable by my anesthesiologist. I have been told and understand that a

small percentage of anesthesia recipients have an allergic or other adverse reaction to the anesthesia they receive and that such reactions, although uncommon, can be serious or fatal.

10. I impose no specific limitations or prohibitions regarding treatment other than those that follow (if none, so state)

_____.

11. I understand that my doctor and other doctors on the staff of this hospital are not employees or agents of the hospital, but are independent contractors who have been granted the privilege of using the hospital facilities for the care and treatment of their patients.

I have read and clearly understand the above and have deleted any portions with which I do not agree. My doctor has fully explained this form to me and answered all my questions. I am satisfied that I understand the content and significance of this form.

_____	_____
Witness	Patient's Signature
	Date: _____ Time: _____

PATIENT CONSENT TO ANESTHESIA

Patient: _____ Date: _____ Time: _____

1. Dr. _____ has told me and I understand that modern anesthesia is relatively safe and uneventful. Most everyone can have the benefits of anesthesia and most operations can be performed with general anesthesia (sodium pentothal by intravenous injection or by inhalation), regional anesthesia (such as epidural, saddle block, spinal, or local), or by a combination of these methods.

2. The specific anesthesia recommended for me is: _____.

3. The doctor has told me and I understand that every type of pain relief has certain risks. Unexpected reactions or complications can occur and their frequency or severity varies between patients even where medical conditions appear otherwise similar.

4. These risks and hazards include, but are not limited to: broken teeth; allergic reactions; pneumonia; phlebitis (inflammation and infection of the veins); nerve injury; paralysis; damage to or failure of the heart, liver, kidneys, and/or brain; and death. These risks and hazards are rare and in most cases anesthesia is administered without any adverse reaction or complication, but no guarantee has been made to me as to the effects on me of the anesthesia to be administered.

5. The doctor has also told me and I understand that at this hospital, anesthesia services are provided by Elekra Medical Group, a private group of physician anesthesiolo-

gists and certified registered nurse anesthetists who work together. This means that the person administering anesthesia to me may not be a physician. However, a physician anesthesiologist will be responsible for the anesthesia services provided to me and will be available in the event his or her services are needed.

6. I consent to the administration of such anesthetics as may be considered necessary or advisable by the physician responsible for administering anesthesia to me, even if such anesthetics differ from those described in paragraph 2, above.

7. I understand that the anesthesia drug or method may be changed, if necessary during the operation or procedure, and consent to whatever anesthesia is chosen by the physician anesthesiologist, with the exception of:

_____

I have read and understand the above and deleted any portions with which I do not agree. The doctor has explained this form to me and answered all my questions. I am satisfied that I understand the content and significance of this form.

_____   _____
Witness   Patient's Signature
                                 Date: _____ Time: _____

CONSENT TO ACCESS TO MEDICAL RECORDS AND RESEARCH PHOTOGRAPHS

Patient: _____ Date: _____ Time: _____

In connection with the medical services which I am receiving from my doctor, Dr._____
_____, he or she has explained to me that he or she or other medical professionals may wish to study my medical records and treatment progress.

I authorize my doctor and the hospital to take photographs or films of me during the course of the treatment and to use such photographs or films together with the information in my medical record, subject to the conditions listed below.

(1) Neither my doctor nor the hospital will identify me by name in the information disclosed from the medical records.

(2) Neither my doctor nor the hospital will use publicly my name or my family's name to identify the photographs or films.

(3) My doctor will disclose the information from the medical records and the photographs or films only for educational or research purposes.

(4) If my doctor believes that medical research, education, or science may benefit by their use, he may authorize the publishing or republishing of the photographs, films, or information relating to my case, either separately or in connection with each other, in professional journals or medical books, or my doctor may authorize any other use which he may deem proper in

the interest of medical education, knowledge, or research.

(5) The photographs or films may be taken only with the consent of my doctor and under such conditions and at such times as he may approve.

(6) I may see the photographs or films if I ask for them.

(7) I can destroy all prints and negatives of the photographs or films if I ask for them in writing.

(8) I may cancel this agreement at any time in writing.

(9) Such additional conditions as follows (if none so state): _____.

I release the hospital, the doctor, and all other persons caring for me or dealing with the records, photographs, or films from all liability resulting from the taking and authorized use of the records, photographs, or films.

I have read and clearly understand the above and have deleted any portions with which I do not agree. The doctor has explained this form to me and answered all my questions. I am satisfied that I understand the content and significance of this form.

_____   _____
Witness   Patient's Signature
                                         Date: _____ Time: _____

PATIENT PASS

Patient: _____ Date: _____ Time: _____

I expect to be away from the hospital from_____
_____ to: _____.

I am leaving the hospital because:_____
_____.

I release the hospital, my physician, and all other persons caring for me from all responsibility for my safety and care and all liability for:

(1) anything happening to me while I am away from the hospital; and

(2) any injury or ill effects resulting from my leaving the hospital.

I understand that Medicare or other insurance may not pay my hospital bill if I go out of the hospital to attend to personal business. I agree to be fully responsible for any portion of the hospital bill not covered by such insurance because I left the hospital. My doctor has warned me

_____
_____.

I have read and clearly understand the above and have deleted any portions with which I do not agree. The doctor has explained this form to me and answered all my questions. I am satisfied that I understand the content and significance of this form.

_____   _____
Witness   Patient's Signature
                          Date: _____ Time: _____

FOR COMPLETION BY THE
ATTENDING PHYSICIAN

I approve the pass requested by this patient for _____ _____ (hours/days). I have examined the patient and I am reasonably certain that it is reasonably safe to permit the patient to be absent from the hospital for this period of time.

_____   _____
Witness   Physician's Signature
                          Date: _____ Time: _____

SIDE RAILS RELEASE

Patient: _____ Date: _____ Time: _____

I understand that side rails are placed on my bed for personal protection. I know that a fall from my bed could result in fractured limbs or vertebrae, brain injury, or other serious bodily injury. Nevertheless, I instruct University Community Hospital, my physician, and all others caring for me NOT to raise the side rails on my bed. I assume all risks and fully release the hospital, my physician, and all others caring for me of all liability for any injury or damage to me caused by the failure to raise the side rails on my bed.

I have read and clearly understand the above and have deleted any portions with which I do not agree. The doctor has explained this form to me and answered all my questions. I am satisfied that I understand the content and significance of this form.

_____   _____
Witness   Patient's Signature
                                Date: _____ Time: _____

PHYSICIAN AUTHORIZATION FOR EMERGENCY TREATMENT FOR ADULT PATIENT

Patient: _____ Date: _____ Time: _____

The patient is unable to give consent to treatment because _____.

Others are not available to give informed consent for the patient because _____.

Searching for other persons to give consent or waiting for the patient to be able to give consent will cause delay which, to a reasonable degree of medical certainty, will result in the patient's death or a serious deterioration of his condition which will endanger his or her health. I believe that immediate treatment is necessary to correct or stabilize the patient's condition, that this treatment is necessary to protect the life or limb of the patient, and that emergency procedures are required.

_____
Physician's Signature
Date: _____ Time: _____ am/pm

SUBSTITUTED GENERAL CONSENT FOR TREATMENT

Patient: _____

Attending Physician: _____

Date of Admission: _____ 19____ Time _____ am/pm
 (or treatment, if outpatient)

1. I authorize University Community Hospital ("the hospital"), its personnel, my doctor, any person under my doctor's direction or responding to his orders, and other professionals with privileges at the hospital to perform all necessary tests and procedures and to administer all necessary medications and treatments required in the course of the diagnosis and treatment of the patient's illness.

2. I am aware that the practice of medicine and surgery is not an exact science and I acknowledge that no guarantees or representations have been made to me as a result of treatments, procedures, or examinations performed or to be performed while I am in the hospital.

3. I consent to the photographing and publication for sale or for medical, scientific, or educational purposes of any all and descriptions, photographs, or videotaping of the operations or procedures to be performed on the patient in the hospital. These photographs and videotapings may include portions of the patient's body, provided the pictures and any descriptive text

accompanying them do not reveal the patient's identity.

4. I authorize the hospital to retain, preserve, use for scientific research, therapeutic or teaching purposes, or dispose of any specimens or tissues taken from the patient's body during the patient's hospitalization.

5. I consent to the release of medical information to other institutions or agencies accepting the patient for medical or institutional care, and consent to the release of medical information to the patient's insurer.

6. I understand that my doctor and other doctors on the staff of this hospital are not employees or agents of the hospital, but are independent contractors who have been granted the privilege of using the hospital facilities for the care and treatment of their patients.

7. I impose no specific limitations or prohibitions regarding treatment other than those that follow (if none, so state):_____

I have read and clearly understand the above and have deleted any portions with which I do not agree. My doctor has fully explained this form to me and answered all my questions. I am satisfied that I understand the content and significance of this form.

The patient is unable to sign and I, as _____ of the patient, hereby consent for the patient.

Witness	Signature
	Date: _____ Time: _____

FOR COMPLETION BY THE ATTENDING PHYSICIAN

The patient is unable to sign because: _____
_____.

_____   _____
Witness   Physician's Signature
                                Date: _____ Time: _____

SUBSTITUTED CONSENT TO OPERATION OR PROCEDURE

Patient: _____ Date: _____ Time: _____

1. After examining the patient, Dr._____
   _____ has told me that the patient has
   _____(name of condition or ailment).

2. The doctor has recommended_____
   _____ (name of operation or procedure). I authorize and consent to the performance upon the patient of this operation or procedure by the doctor and any assistants, including hospital personnel, supervised by him who he believes are necessary and appropriate.

3. I have discussed with the doctor the following issues summarized below. The doctor has explained these issues to me, answered all my questions, and I understand that:

   A. The nature and purpose of the operation or procedure is:_____
      _____.

   B. The risks and benefits of the operation or procedure are: _____
      _____.

   C. The possible or likely consequences of the procedure are: _____
      _____.

   D. The alternatives methods of treatment are:_____
      _____
      _____.

Sample Consent Forms

E. The risks and benefits of these alternatives are:_____
_____
_____.

F. The risks of refusing treatment entirely are:_____
_____
_____.

4. The doctor has told me and I understand that during the course of the operation or procedure, unforeseen conditions may require additional or different procedures than set forth above. I authorize and request that my doctor and his assistants perform such procedures as my doctor believes are necessary.

5. I acknowledge that no guarantee or assurance has been given by anyone as to the results or outcome of, or recovery from, these operations or procedures.

6. For the purpose of advancing medical education, I consent to the admittance of observers to the room where the operation or procedure is to be performed.

7. I hereby authorize University Community Hospital to retain, preserve, use for scientific research, therapeutic, or teaching purposes, or dispose of any specimens or tissues taken from the patient's body during hospitalization except as specified below (if none so state):_____
_____.

8. I agree that the patient receive blood or blood products or derivatives as deemed necessary by my doctor. I have been told and understand that a small percentage of blood recipients have an allergic or other adverse reaction to the blood they receive and that such reactions, although rare, can be serious or fatal.

9. I consent to the administration of anesthesia to be applied by or under the direction of an anesthesiologist and to the use of anesthetics he may deem desirable. I also consent to the administration of anesthesia different from that planned if it is considered necessary or advisable by my anesthesiologist. I have been told and understand that a small percentage of anesthesia recipients have an allergic or other adverse reaction to the anesthesia they receive and that such reactions, although uncommon, can be serious or fatal.

10. I impose no specific limitations or prohibitions regarding treatment other than those that follow (if none, so state)

_____
_____.

11. I understand that my doctor and other doctors on the staff of this hospital are not employees or agents of the hospital, but are independent contractors who have been granted the privilege of using the hospital facilities for the care and treatment of their patients.

I have read and clearly understand the above and have deleted any portions with which I do not agree. My doctor has fully explained this form to me and answered all my questions. I am satisfied that I understand the content and significance of this form.

The patient is unable to sign and I, as _____ of the patient, hereby consent for the patient.

_____   _____
Witness   Signature
                                                       Date: _____ Time: _____

FOR COMPLETION BY THE ATTENDING PHYSICIAN

The patient is unable to sign because:_____

_____

_____   _____
Witness   Physician's Signature
                              Date: _____ Time: _____

SUBSTITUTED CONSENT TO ANESTHESIA

Patient: _____ Date: _____ Time: _____

1. Dr. _____ has told me and I understand that modern anesthesia is relatively safe and uneventful. Most everyone can have the benefits of anesthesia and most operations can be performed with general anesthesia (sodium pentothal by intravenous injection or by inhalation), regional anesthesia (such as epidural, saddle block, spinal, or local), or by a combination of these methods.

2. The specific anesthesia recommended for the patient is:_____ .

3. The doctor has told me and I understand that every type of pain relief has certain risks. Unexpected reactions or complications can occur and their frequency or severity varies between patients even where medical conditions appear otherwise similar.

4. These risks and hazards include, but are not limited to: broken teeth; allergic reactions; pneumonia; phlebitis (inflammation and infection of the veins); nerve injury; paralysis; damage to or failure of the heart, liver, kidneys, and/or brain; and death. These risks and hazards are rare and in most cases anesthesia is administered without any adverse reaction or complication, but no guarantee has been made to me as to the effects on the patient of the anesthesia to be administered.

5. The doctor has also told me and I understand that at this hospital, anesthesia services are provided by Elekra Medical Group, a private group of physician anesthesiolo-

Sample Consent Forms

gists and certified registered nurse anesthetists who work together. This means that the person administering anesthesia to the patient may not be a physician. However, a physician anesthesiologist will be responsible for the anesthesia services provided to the patient and will be available in the event his or her services are needed.

6. I consent to the administration of such anesthetics as may be considered necessary or advisable by the physician responsible for administering anesthesia to the patient, even if such anesthetics differ from those described in paragraph 2, above.

7. I understand that the anesthesia drug or method may be changed, if necessary during the operation or procedure, and consent to whatever anesthesia is chosen by the physician anesthesiologist, with the exception of:_____ _____.

I have read and understand the above and deleted any portions with which I do not agree. The doctor has explained this form to me and answered all my questions. I am satisfied that I understand the content and significance of this form.

The patient is unable to sign and I, as_____ of the patient, hereby consent for the patient.

_____	_____
Witness	Signature
	Date: _____ Time: _____

**FOR COMPLETION BY THE
ATTENDING PHYSICIAN**

The patient is unable to sign because: _____
_____.

_____   _____
Witness   Physician's Signature
                                                Date: _____ Time: _____

Notes

1. This consent policy is adopted from the University Community Hospital Consent in Florida consent policy as developed by Carlton, Fields, Ward, Emmanuel, Smith & Cutler, P.A., Attorneys at Law, Tampa, Florida. It was prepared on the basis of Florida statutes and appellate court decisions and obviously should be used as a guide to areas to be covered only as other states have different requirements and Florida law may have changed by the time this book is published. Consultation with a healthcare attorney before adopting a consent policy is a must.

2. Again, these consent forms are for a specific Florida hospital and may not be sufficient for other hospitals within or without that state.

Glossary

Actual damages—Damages awarded for a loss or injury the plaintiff really suffered.

Battery—Both a crime and a tort consisting of an unconsented harmful or offensive touching.

Battery consent form—A document that authorizes a procedure but does not contain sufficient details as to the consequences, risks, and alternatives of the proposed treatment to protect against a lack of informed consent claim.

Blanket consent form—A document that purports to authorize any and all procedures.

Competent—Legally qualified or able.

Emancipation—The legal doctrine that allows a minor to act as an adult when he or she has moved away from home and receives no support for his or her parents.

Emergency exception—The legal doctrine that excuses failure to obtain consent when the patient requires immediate treatment and unable to give consent and the physician cannot obtain substituted consent in a timely fashion.

Federal Tort Claims Act—The federal law that makes the United States liable for the acts and omissions of its officers and employees occurring within the scope of their employment.

Good Samaritan Statute—A law that immunizes one who provides emergency medical care from liability unless they were grossly negligent or intentionally injured the patient.

Guardian—A person appointed by a court to manage and control a person who is not competent to manage his or her own affairs.

Incompetent—One who is unable or unfit to make decisions.

Independent contractor—The opposite of an employee—one hired to do a specific task, the detailed performance of which is not controlled by the entity hiring the independent contractor. A healthcare entity is generally not liable for the acts of independent contractors it utilizes.

Informed consent—The tort doctrine, based on the negligent failure of a physician to disclose to a patient information that would enable the patient to evaluate knowledgeably the treatment options and risks before consenting to the treatment.

Intentional tort—A deliberate or purposeful civil wrong as opposed to a negligent one.

Living will—A legal document executed when a person is competent specifying that certain type of medical care be discontinued if the patient becomes incompetent and terminally ill or in an irreversible coma.

Negligence—The tort of harming another by a failure to use due care.

Parens patriae **power**—A state's power to supervise minors and those under a legally disability to assure their welfare.

Prognosis—A predication about the probable outcome of a disease or injury.

Punitive damages—Damages over and above actual damages that are designed to punish a tortfeasor.

Reasonable patient standard—The legal doctrine that specifies that a physician's duty to disclose in informed consent cases is measured by the materiality of the information to the patient's decision.

Reasonable physician standard—The legal doctrine that specifies that a physician's duty to disclose in informed consent cases is limited to those disclosures which a reasonable medical practitioner would make under the same or similar circumstances.

Substituted consent—Consent from a person authorized to decide on behalf of an incompetent or incapacitated patient.

Therapeutic privilege—An exception to the rule requiring informed consent in cases in which full disclosure would harm the patient.

Tort—A civil, as opposed to a criminal, wrong. A tort subjects the tortfeasor to liability for damages caused by the wrong.

Tortfeasor—One who commits a civil wrong.

Bibliography

American Medical Association. *Current Opinions of the Council on Ethical and Judicial Affairs of the American Medical Association*. Chicago, IL: American Medical Association, 1989, § 5.05.

Centers for Disease Control. *Recommendations for Prevention of HIV Transmission in Health-Care Settings*. 36 MMWR, Supp. No. 2S, Aug. 21, 1987, 15S.

Department of Health, Education and Welfare. *The Institutional Guide to DHEW Policy on Protection of Human Subjects*, DHEW Publication No. 72-102. Washington D.C.: U.S. Government Printing Office No. 1740-0326, December 1971.

Barry R. Furrow, Sandra H. Johnson, Timothy S. Jost, & Robert L. Schwartz. *Health Law, Cases, Materials and Problems*, 2d ed. St. Paul, Minn.: West Publishing Co., 1991.

Terese Hudson. "Informed Consent Problems Become More Complicated." *Hospitals 1991* 65, No. 6 (March 20, 1991), 38-40.

II Hospital Law Manual. Rockville, Md.: Aspen Systems Corp. December 1982, 52-53.

Joint Commission on Accreditation of Healthcare Organizations. *Accreditation Manual for Hospitals, 1991* xiii (1990).

Theodore LeBlang & W. Eugene Basanta. *The Law of Medical Practice in Illinois*. Rochester, N.Y.: Lawyer's Co-operative Publishing Co. 1986.

Dennis Moloney. *Protection of Human Research Subjects: A Practical Guide to Federal Laws and Regulations.* New York: Plenum Press 1984.

R. Miller. *Problems in Hospital Law*, 6th ed. Rockville, Md.: Aspen Systems Corp. 1990.

Arnold J. Rosoff. *Informed Consent.* Rockville, Md.: Aspen Systems Corp. 1981.

Fay A. Rozovsky. *Consent to Treatment*, 2d ed. Boston, Toronto & London: Little, Brown & Co. 1984 & 1991 Supp.

Richard E. Shugrue & Kathyrn Linstromberg. "Practitioner's Guide to Informed Consent." *Creighton Law Review* 24 (1990-91), 881.

Ron Winslow. "Sometimes Talk is the Best Medicine: For Physicians, Communications May Avert Suits." *Wall Street Journal* (October 5, 1989), B1.

Index

A

Abortion, 39, 84, 85, 91-96, 112, 117
  see Emergency, Nonemergency
Action, *see* Battery, Malpractice
Admission, 27
AIDS, 34, 35, 89
  testing, 33, 38-39, 69, 93
  virus infection, 88
Alabama
  hospital(s), 72
  informed consent law, 69-70
  Supreme Court, 69
Alaska informed consent law, 70-71
Alternative(s), 30, 37, 47, 83, 94, 106, 107, 114
  see Diagnosis, Procedure, Reasonable
  method, 65
  procedure(s), 79, 90
  treatment, 44, 47, 76, 90
American Hospital Association, 5
Amputation, 20
Anatomical gifts, 104
Anesthesia, 29, 30, 112
  see Patient Consent to Anesthesia, Substituted Consent
  Consent, 112
Anesthesiologist, 112
Anguish, *see* Mental
Antagonist drug, 90

Appendices, 111-144
Arbiter, 4
Arizona
  informed consent law, 71
  statutes, 71
Arkansas
  informed consent law, 71-72
  statute, 71
Arteriograms, 112
Arthritis, 14
Artificial insemination, 39
Attending physician, 105
Attorney, *see* Healthcare, Power
Authorization, 8
  see Physician, State
Authorized
  persons, 8-10
  representative, 77
Autopsy, 32, 36-37, 104

B

Battery, 2-3, 8, 21, 28, 105
  action, 76
  consent forms, 106-107
  liability, 53-54
Benefit(s), 46, 76, 81, 87, 94, 107, 114
  see Organ, Procedure
  doctrine, 57
Bibliography, 149-150
Birth defects, 39

Blanket
   admission consent forms, 106
   consent forms, 106
Blood, 33, 38
   donations, 32, 34-35
   drawing, 35
   serum, 33
   test, 38
   testing, 78, 94
   transfusion, 13, 32, 34-35, 59
Blood-borne infectious disease, 78-79
Bodily fluids, 94
Body parts use, 32, 33-34
Bone marrow aspirate, 33
Brain damage, 29, 79
Breast
   cancer treatment, 87
   disease, 91
   tumor treatment, 95

C

California
   Civic Code, 72
   informed consent law, 72
   Supreme Court, 33
Cancer, 30
   see Breast cancer treatment
Cardiac/respiratory arrest, 20
Care, 66
Cataract extraction, 54
Causation, 56, 83, 87
Center for Disease Control (CDC), 38
Chemotherapy, 13, 32, 112
Claims, 5
Coercion, *see* Express, Implied
Colorado
   hospital(s), 72
   informed consent law, 72-73
Commercial development, 33
Common
   law, *see* Federal
   risk, 70

Compensation, 19, 62
Complication, 76, 89
   see Surgery
Confidential treatment, 39
Confidentiality, *see* Records
Confirmatory testing, 39
Connecticut
   commissioner of mental retardation, 73
   informed consent law, 73
Consent
   see Anesthesia, Expressed, Facility, Federal, General, Implied, Informed, Louisiana, Minor, Parental, Patient Consent, Refusal, Special, State, Substituted, Treatment, Uniform, Uninformed
   decision, 90
   forms, 105-109
      see Battery, Blanket, Detailed, Emergency, Nonemergency, Non-English
   samples, 121-144
   process, 108
   withdrawal right, 82
   withholding, 76, 80, 93
Consent to Operation or Procedure, 112
Consent policy, 32
   see Facility, Legally
   forms, 111-113
   procedures, 113-120
   samples, 111-120
   specifications, 104-105
Consent for Treatment and Release of Information by Patient, 121-123
Consenter, qualification, 7-24
Consultation, 116, 118
Contract(s), *see* Department of Health and Human Services
Contractor, *see* Independent

Corporation responsibility, 57
Counseling services, 77

D

D&C, *see* Dilation
Damages, 53, 54, 74, 83
  see Punitive
Death, 46, 79, 118
  risk, 36, 47
Deception, 80, 88
Defendant, 3
  see Physician/defendant
Delaware
  informed consent definition, 73
  informed consent law, 73-74
Department of Health and Human Services, 31, 61
  contracts, 64
  grants, 31, 64
  HHS, 31, 61, 64, 65
  rules, 64
Dependent, *see* Minor
Detailed consent forms, 107-109
Development, 31, 33
Diabetes, 20
Diagnosis, 46, 59, 74, 87, 94
  alternatives, 91
Diagnostic
  procedures, 27, 46, 112
  test, 46
Dilation and curettage (D&C), 28
Diligence, 69
Disability, 37, 46, 47
  see Legal
Disclosure, 76, 89, 90
  see Information, Patient, Reasonable, Risk
  duty, 71
  requirements, 82
  standard, 45-46, 57, 92
Discomfort, 47
Discrimination, 38
Disease, 118
  see Health-threatening, Life-threatening
Disfigurement, 47
Disfiguring scar, 79
Doctor-patient relationship, 3-4
Documentation, 105, 118
Donation, *see* Blood, Organ
Donee, 37
Donor, 37
Drug(s), 113
  see Antagonist, Experimental
  abuse, 117
  dependency, 90
  therapy, 32

E

Elective procedure, 46, 50
Electroconvulsive therapy, 29, 31, 112
Emancipated minor, 117
Embryo, 63
Emergency, 49-50, 89, 91
  see Nonemergency
  abortion, 119
  care, 20, 58
  exceptions, 19-22, 50
  medical treatment, 49, 118
  room/room care, 58
  setting, 86
  situation, 55
    consent forms, 118-119
  treatment, *see* Physician Authorization
Employee, 57
  relationship, 57
Ethical integrity, 18
Ethics committee, 15
Evaluation, 94
Examination
  see Proposed
  outcome, 77
Exceptions, 64
Excision, 108
Experimental
  drugs, 64

medical research, 77
procedures, 29, 31, 62, 112
research, 95-96
therapy, 78
treatment, 77
Experimentation, *see* Fetal, Human, Infant, Maternal
Express coercion, 81
Expressed consent, 27

F

Facility
  consent policies, 59-60, 103-110
  liability, practitioner obtainment failure, 57-59
  policy, 37
FDA, *see* Food and Drug Administration
Federal
  common law, 61
  hospitals, 61
  informed consent laws, 61-67
    guidance, 65-66
  laws, 64
  Tort Claims Act (FTCA), 61
Fetal experimentation, 86, 91
Fetus, 39, 63
Fiduciary obligation, 33
Findings, 63
Florida
  informed consent law, 74-75
  Medical Consent Law, 74
Follow-up care, 37
Food and Drug Administration, 61
  FDA, 61, 62, 64
  rules, 64
Fraud, 80, 88
FTCA, *see* Federal Tort

G

General Consent, *see* Substituted
General Consent for Treatment, 111
Georgia
  informed consent law, 75-76
  statutes, 44
Glossary, 145-147
Good Samaritan, 19
Grant(s), *see* Department of Health and Human Services
Gross negligence, 19
Guardian, 9, 11, 15, 35, 76, 115, 117, 119

H

Hairy-cell leukemia, 33
Hawaii
  Board of Medical Examiners, 76
  Code, 76
  informed consent law, 76
Healthcare
  attorney, 50
  delivery, supervision, 59
  facility, 27, 82, 90
  institutions, 58
  law, 57
  practitioner, 9
  profession, 88
  providers, 7, 8, 10, 18-21, 31, 44, 45, 70, 73, 80, 92, 93, 95
  services, 90
  surrogates, 75
  treatment, 4
Health-threatening
  condition, 50
  disease/injury, 49
Hepatitis, 34, 78
  B testing, 83
HHS, *see* Department of Health and Human Services
Hiatal hernia, 21, 22
High-risk group, 34
HIV, 34, 35, 38
  antibody, 38
  infection, 78
  informed consent, *see* Uniform
  testing, 38, 70, 72-78, 80, 81, 83, 84, 86-89, 95, 96, 105, 113

Hormone treatments, 112
Hospital
 see Alabama, Colorado, Federal, Joint
 employee, 114
 liability, 57-59
 patient, 81
 personnel, 112
 procedures, 106
Human
 experimentation, 91, 104
 research, 95
 research review committee, 87

I
Idaho informed consent law, 76-77
Illinois
 informed consent law, 77
 Mental Health Code, 30-31
Immediate consent, 50
Implied
 coercion, 81
 consent, 27
In loco parentis, 9
Infant experimentation, 86
Incapacitation, 86, 88, 94
Incision, 112
Incompetent patient, 14-18, 104
Independent contractor, 57-59
 practitioner, 57
Indiana informed consent law, 77-78
Information, 71, 77, 96
 see Consent for Treatment, Patient, Risk
Information disclosure, 72, 79
 amount, 46-47
 nondisclosure, 47-48
 physician, 43-45
 risks, 46
Informed consent
 see Delaware, Federal, Research, State, Treatment, Uniform, Uninformed, Written
 additional elements, 63-64
 basic elements, 62-63
 claims, 5
 definition, 1-6
 doctrine, 8
 importance, 1-6
 obtainment process, 43-51
 obtainment failure, 3-4
  see Facility
 liability, 53-60
 special situations, 32-39
 standard, 82
 timing, 27-41
 user, 7-24
Informed participation, 59
Injured
 party, 74
 person, 71, 72
Injury, 62, 85, 93, 95
 see Health-threatening, Life-threatening, Plaintiff, Research-related, Sudden
Inoculations, 32, 34
Institutional
 review, 61
 Review Board (IRB), 65
Insurance, 38
Intentional
 act, 2
 invasion, 54
 misconduct, 19
 tort, 2
Intervention, 36
Intoxicants, 113
Intraocular lens implant, 54
Invasion, see Intentional, Patient
Invasive procedures, 112
 see Nonsurgical
Investigator, 63
Iowa informed consent law, 78
IRB, see Institutional Review Board

J
Jehovah's Witness, 35

Joint Commission on Accreditation of Healthcare Organizations, 65, 105
Joint Commission on the Accreditation of Hospitals, 58, 59
Judicial scrutiny, 107
Jurisdictions, 48
Jury, 56, 59, 91
Juvenile court, 117

K
Kansas
 informed consent law, 78
 Supreme Court, 43
Kentucky informed consent law, 78-78
Ketoacidosis, 20

L
Laetrile use, 96
Law(s), 59
 see Common, Federal, Federal common, Local, State
Lawsuit, 53
Legal
 disability, 12
 guardians, 5
 representative, 64, 111, 114
Legally sufficient consent policy, 103-105
Leukemia, 13
 see Hairy-cell
Liability, 3, 4, 19, 59, 72, 103, 109
 see Battery, Facility, Hospital, Informed, Malpractice, Risk
 immunity, 57
 limit, 80
Life-saving treatment, 36, 112
Life-sustaining
 medical treatment, 15, 16, 18
 treatment, 18
Life-threatening
 condition, 50
 disease/injury, 49
 situation, 64
Living will, 15, 16
Lobotomies, 112
Local laws, 64
Louisiana
 informed consent law, 79-80
 Uniform Consent Law, 28
Low-risk procedure, 35

M
Maine
 informed consent law, 80-81
 statute, 80
Malpractice, 4, 54, 59, 71
 action, 92
 liability, 109
Maryland informed consent law, 81
Massachusetts informed consent law, 81-82
Material
 facts, 89, 95
 issues, 107
 risk, 77, 78, 90, 91
Maternal experimentation, 86
Medicaid, 65
Medical
 care provider, 71, 72
 community, 47, 48
 emergencies, 19, 21-22
 judgment, 113
 malpractice, 2, 8
 practice, accepted standard, 75, 79
 procedures, 1, 78
 records, 48, 107, 114, 116
  see Consent to Access
 research, *see* Experimental
 risk, 86
 services, 88, 117
 standard, 70
 technology, 5
 test, 78
 testimony, 45, 56, 91

treatment, 7-11, 14, 16, 17, 19, 21, 33, 62, 79, 92, 117
see Emergency, Life-sustaining
Medicare, 65
Mental
  anguish, 54
  illness, 113
    see Nonemergency treatment
  health facilities, 75
Michigan informed consent law, 82
Midwife, 84
Minimal risk, 62, 64
Minnesota
  informed consent law, 82-83
  statutes, 83
Minor(s), 84, 91, 104, 117, 118-119
  see Emancipated, Unwed
  care, 72
  child, 8
  consent, 11
  dependent, 36
  patients, 10-14, 30
  pregnant women, 93
Misconduct, *see* Intentional
Misrepresentation, 75, 79, 80, 88, 89
Mississippi
  Code, 83
  informed consent law, 83
Missouri informed consent law, 84
Montana informed consent law, 84
Myelograms, 112

N

Nebraska informed consent law, 84-85
Negligence, 3, 29, 53, 54, 57-59, 61, 79, 84, 93
  see Gross
  actions, 54, 56
  concept, 1
  definition, 54-55
  law principles, 55
  theory, 2
Nevada
  informed consent law, 85
  statutes, 85
New Hampshire
  informed consent law, 85-86
  Supreme Court, 87
New Jersey
  Bill of Rights, 86
  informed consent law, 86
New Mexico informed consent law, 86-87
New York
  informed consent law, 87
  Public Health Law, 87
  statute limits, 87
Nondisclosure, 49, 105
  see Information
Nonemergency
  abortion, 117
  situations, consent form, 115-117
  surgery, 87
  treatment, 74, 87
    mental illness, 76
Non-English speaking patients, consent forms, 119-120
Nonsurgical
  invasive procedures, 32
  procedures, 112
Nontreatment, 76
  religious motivation, 32, 35-36
North Carolina
  informed consent law, 87-88
  statutes, 87
North Dakota informed consent law, 88-89
Nurse practitioner, 105
Nursing home, 66, 95
  patient, 77

O

Objective
  approach, 15
  test, 56
Obligation, *see* Fiduciary
OBRA, see Omnibus Budget Rec-

oncilation Act
Ohio informed consent law, 89
Oklahoma
  informed consent law, 89-90
  judicial opinions, 90
  statutes, 89
Ominibus Budget Reconciliation
    Act (OBRA), 66
One-patient treatment, 37
Operation, 32, 54, 113
  see Patient Consent, Substituted
    Consent
Option, 1
Oregon informed consent law, 90
Organ donation, 33, 37
  risk/benefit, 37

P

Paralysis, 46
  risk, 29
Paraplegia, 29, 79
Parens patriae, 12, 13
Parental
  consent, 10, 11
  permission, 59
Participation, 62, 63
  see Social Security Act
  termination, 63
Patent, 33
Pathological assessment, 108
Patient
  see Consent for Treatment, Doctor-patient, Hospital, Incompetent, Minor, Non-English, Nursing home, Physician Authorization, Physician-patient, Provider-patient, Reasonable
  alternative methods, 85
  condition, 77
  information, 88
    disclosure, 111
  need to know, 90
  objection, 35
  participation, 1
  Pass, 131-132
  privacy invasion, 32, 34
  signature, 105
Patient Consent to Anesthesia, 127-128
Patient Consent to Operation or
    Procedure, 124-126
Patient/plaintiff, 55, 56, 71, 84, 85
Pennsylvania informed consent
    law, 90-91
Permission, 59
Pharmaceutical research, 74
Photographs, 32, 34
  see Consent to Access, Research
Physician, 1-3, 7, 27, 28, 32-34, 37,
    46, 48, 53, 72, 78, 81, 83, 90,
    91, 95, 104, 116
  see Attending, Information, Reasonable, Treating
  judgment, 111
Physician Authorization for Emergency Treatment for Adult
    Patient, 134
Physician/defendant, 56, 84
Physician-patient relationship, 55
Plaintiff, 2, 3, 30, 33, 34, 53, 55, 56,
    58, 84
  see Patient/plaintiff
  condition, 57
  injury, 55
Podiatrist, 91
Policy for Withholding Treatment,
    115
Post-treatment therapy, 16
Power of attorney, 15
Practitioners, 4, 7, 28, 30, 37, 38,
    43, 46, 47, 50, 57, 69, 75, 76,
    80, 82, 88, 92, 94, 103, 107
  see Facility, Independent, Nurse,
    Reasonable
Pregnancy, 36, 63, 117, 119
  termination, 116

Privacy
  see Patient
  right, 18, 34
Procedure(s), 28, 29, 32, 48, 113
  see Alternative, Consent policy, Diagnostic, Experimental, Hospital, Low-risk, Medical, Patient Consent, Proposed, Substituted Consent, Therapeutic, Unauthorized
  alternatives, 73
  benefits, 47, 73
  outcome, 77
  risks, 73
Professional services, 69
Prognosis, 16, 17, 59
Proposed
  examination, 77
  procedures, 44, 70, 73, 77, 85, 91
  therapy, 46, 88
  treatment, 44, 46, 70, 73, 77, 79, 80, 88, 91, 95
Providers, 71, 74, 79
  see Healthcare, Medical
Provider-patient relationship, 93
Proximate cause, 55
Prudent person, 56
Psychological
  distress, 38
  risk, 86
Psychosurgery, 116
Psychotropic medication, 92
Punitive damages, 3, 54
Pyelograms, 112

Q
Quadraplegia, 29, 79

R
Radiation therapy, 30-31
Radiological therapy, 29, 112
Radiologist, 29, 58
Reasonable
  alternatives, 70, 94, 108
  care, 69
  disclosure, 43-44, 88, 91, 92
  individual, 79
  medical practitioner, 45
  patient, 45, 55-56, 73
    standard, 48, 55
  person, 44-45, 75, 80, 88, 93, 94
  physician standard, 45-46, 47, 55
    jurisdiction, 55
  practitioners, 55, 84, 97
  treatment alternative(s), 78
Records
  see Consent to Access, Medical
  confidentiality, 62
Recuperation, 37, 46, 108
Referral, 77
Refusal to consent, 17
Release, *see* Consent for Treatment, Side Rails
Religious beliefs, 36
Remission, 13
Representative, *see* Authorized, Legal
Reproductive matters, 33, 39-40, 104
Research, 31, 33, 64
  see Experimental, Medical, Pharmaceutical
  acceptability, 65
  informed consent, 61-65
  photographs, *see* Consent to Access
  proposals, 65
  withdrawal, 63
Research-related injury, 63
Retention, 32, 33-34
Rheumatic fever, 14
Rhode Island informed consent law, 91
Risk, 1, 2, 4, 12, 27-31, 33, 34, 43-48, 62, 63, 70, 71, 76, 79-81, 83, 85, 87, 88, 91, 93, 94, 96, 107, 112, 114

see Common, Death, High-risk, Material, Medical, Minimal, Organ, Paralysis, Procedure, Psychological, Test, Treatment
  disclosure, 74, 80
    failure, 79
  information, 55
  liability, 8
  management, 5
Routine testing, 38
Rule of Sevens, 10

S

Scar(s), 47
  see Disfiguring
Scarring, 37
Sexual function impairment, 37
Side effects, 16, 32
Side Rails Release, 133
Social Security Act
  Conditions of Participation, 65
  section 1865, 65
Sodium pentothal, 30
South Carolina informed consent law, 91-92
South Dakota
  informed consent law, 92
  statutes, 92
Special Consent, 112
Staff, 58
  supervision, 57
Standard
  see Disclosure, Medical, Reasonable
  of care, 53, 54
  practice, 45
Standardized written consent, 87
State
  authorization, 11-14
  informed consent laws, 69-102
    see also individual states
  interests, 17
  laws, 64

Statutes, 3, 8, 36, 38, 69, 70, 103, 104
  see also individual states
Sterilization, 90, 95, 104, 112, 116, 117
Subjective test, 56
Substituted
  consent, 7, 8, 14, 50, 72, 85, 92, 114
  Consent to Anesthesia, 142-144
  Consent to Operation or Procedure, 138-141
  decision maker, 17
  General Consent for Treatment, 135-137
  judgment, 15
Success
  probability, 47
  rate, 47
Sudden injury, 19, 20
Suicide, 36
Supervision, *see* Healthcare, Staff
Supreme Court, *see* Alabama, California, Kansas, New Mexico, United States
Surgery, 1, 3, 28, 29, 34, 35, 84, 87, 96, 112
  see Nonemergency, Psychosurgery, Tear
  complications, 57
Surgical
  procedure, 28, 76, 89
  services, 117
  treatment, 19
  wound infection, 84

T

Tear duct surgery, 54
Technology, see Medical
Tennessee informed consent law, 92-93
Termination, *see* Participation
Test, 81, 113
  see Blood, Confirmatory, Diag-

nostic, Medical, Objective, Subjective
administration, 82
availability, 39
explanation, 82
outcome, 77
participation, 82
results, 81
  confidentiality, 82
  disclosure, 38-39
risk, 39
Testimony, *see* Medical
Testing, *see* Blood, HIV
Texas informed consent law, 93
Therapeutic
privilege, 48-49, 50
procedures, 27
Therapy, *see* Chemotherapy, Drug, Electroconvulsive, Experimental, Proposed, Radiation, Radiological
success probability, 81
Thrombophlebitis, 20
T-lymphocytes, 33
Tort, 57
see Federal Tort, Intentional
Touching, *see* Unauthorized
Treating physician, 105
Treatment
see Breast tumor, Confidential, Consent for Treatment, Experimental, Immediate, Information, Life-saving, Medical, Nonemergency, Nontreatment, One-patient, Physician Authorization, Policy, Post-treatment, Proposed, Reasonable, Substituted, Surgical, Unauthorized
alternatives, 47, 73, 91, 96
consequences, 78
decision, 48, 49
outcome, 77

record, 49
refusal, 96
religious motivation, 32, 35-36
requiring consent, 27-28
requiring informed consent, 28-32
risks, 19, 44, 46, 73, 75

U
Unauthorized
procedure, 53-54, 59
touching, 28, 53, 105
treatment, 28
Unconsciousness, 72
Uniform
consent, *see* Louisiana
written HIV informed consent, 81
Uninformed consent, 49
United States
Constitution, 40
Supreme Court, 10
Unprofessional conduct, 78
Unwed minor mother, 117
Utah informed consent law, 93-94

V
Venereal disease, 89, 117
Vermont
informed consent definition, 94
informed consent law, 94
statute, 94
Vexicovaginal fistula, 28
Violence, 36
Virginia informed consent law, 95

W
Waivers, 64
Washington
informed consent law, 95-96
statutes, 95
West Virginia
Code, 96
informed consent law, 96
Wisconsin informed consent law, 96

Withholding, *see* Consent, Policy
Witness credibility, 91
Written
  confirmation, 114
  consent, 77, 79
    see Standardized, Uniform
  consent to treatment, 75
  informed consent, 38, 74, 95
Wyoming informed consent law,
    97

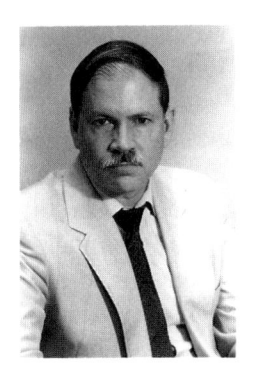

About the Author

Jonathan P. Tomes is an associate professor at IIT Chicago-Kent College of Law. Among the subjects he has taught is administrative law—the part of the law that deals with the rules and regulations that administrative agencies, such as the Environmental Protection Agency, Health and Human Services, the Occupational Safety and Health Administration, and so forth, issue to control publicly regulated businesses such as healthcare providers and hospital law.

Before going to law school, Professor Tomes served as an infantry platoon leader in Vietnam, where he won the Silver Star and the Combat Infantry Badge among other awards. Then he graduated first in his class at Oklahoma City University School of Law and won the Oklahoma Bar Association outstanding law student award. He is a member of the Illinois and Oklahoma bars. Following graduation, he served in the Judge Advocate General's Corps, U.S. Army, until he retired as a lieutenant colonel in 1988. While in the military, he served as prosecutor, defense counsel, and military judge before becoming Chief of Special Claims, Tort Claims Division, U.S. Army Claims Service, where he was in charge of processing and adjudicating claims that occurred overseas against the military, primarily medical malpractice claims. That assignment led to his interest in healthcare law. The military rewarded his 20 years' service by awarding him the Legion of Merit, the second-highest service award in the military, upon his retirement.

Among Professor Tomes's publications are *The Servicemember's Legal Guide, Healthcare Records: A Practical Legal Guide,* three books for the HFMA Trustee's Guide series, *Understanding Healthcare Environmental Law, Understanding Healthcare Antitrust Law, Understanding Medical Staff Privilege,* and four other books for Probus Publishing's Guide for the Healthcare Professional series, *Environmental Law, Antitrust Law, Fraud & Abuse Laws and Safe Harbors,* and *Regulation of the Healthcare Industry* as well as articles in the *Boston University Annual Review of Banking Law, Richmond Law Review, Air Force Law Review* (the U.S. Supreme Court cited his article in this law review), *Association Management* and *The Practical Lawyer.*

About the Publisher

PROBUS PUBLISHING COMPANY

Probus Publishing Company fills the informational needs of today's business professional by publishing authoritative, quality books on timely and relevant topics, including:

- Investing
- Futures/Options Trading
- Banking
- Finance
- Marketing and Sales
- Manufacturing and Project Management
- Personal Finance, Real Estate, Insurance and Estate Planning
- Entrepreneurship
- Management

Probus books are available at quantity discounts when purchased for business, educational or sales promotional use. For more information, please call the Director, Corporate/Institutional Sales at 1-800-998-4644, or write:

Director, Corporate/Institutional Sales
Probus Publishing Company
1925 N. Clybourn Avenue
Chicago, Illinois 60614
FAX (312) 868-6250